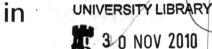

The NH...ct

The biggest ... imme in ...

Sea...

Radcliffe Publishing

Oxford • Seattle

Radcliffe Publishing Ltd
18 Marcham Road
Abingdon
Oxon OX14 1AA
United Kingdom

www.radcliffe-oxford.com
Electronic catalogue and worldwide online ordering facility.

British Library Cataloguing in Publication Data

A catalogue record for this book is available from the British Library.

ISBN 10: 1 85775 732 7
ISBN 13: 978 1 85775 732 3

Typeset by Anne Joshua & Associates, Oxford
Printed and bound by TJI Digital, Padstow, Cornwall

Contents

Preface

Early in the spring of 2003, the National Health Service in England placed a series of abstruse, technically worded, advertisements into the Appendices of the Official Journal of the European Communities.

This is a publication referred to normally by its acronym – 'OJEC'. You won't have seen this journal on the bookstands. It is an esoteric, magazine-sized document, published every day, and read only by the marketing boffins of big corporations. There are no features or articles to distract the reader. It consists of nothing more than curious, numbered lists, painstakingly documenting every major public procurement within the borders of Europe. Here are invitations to participate in huge procurements: battleships for the Spanish Navy, underpants for the Greek Army, tarmac for German autobahns, felt pens for Swedish schools.

The NHS advertisements did not stand out among this maelstrom of official business. Yet this was the start of what was destined to become the single biggest IT project in world history, galvanising tens of thousands of people, and consuming billions of pounds of taxpayers' money. The conclusion of this project will be nothing less than a wholesale reinvention of the way that healthcare is managed and delivered in England. It will put new tools into the hands of doctors and nurses that will change their lives as care givers, and may even save our lives as patients.

The biggest computer programme in the world ever? Surely not! Wasn't there a huge American Army computer programme? An integrated procurement and logistics programme which provides complete lifecycle management of every component used in the military and aerospace industry in the US? Doesn't it cover design right through from component to full system, manufacture, procurement, shipping, installation, maintenance and disposal?

Possibly. But was it really bigger than the medical records of over 50 million people? Did it really have as wide a reach of applications as a system that will daily log the results of several million blood tests, that will hold millions of X-ray images, that will track the movements of millions of sets of patient notes, that will communicate hundreds of thousands of prescriptions? More significantly, will it be used continuously right through the working day by more than half a million demanding users?

When we use the words 'biggest' or 'largest' it can often come down to definition. Which is the world's largest airport? King Khalid International Airport in Riyadh, Saudi Arabia takes some beating. It takes up some 81 square miles. But by another measure, Atlanta Hartsfield Jackson is the busiest airport in the world, handling 76.7 million passengers in 2002, more than any other airport. When the flights from all airports in a city are combined, London is the busiest aviation centre in the world, busier even than New York or Tokyo. So which is the busiest airport in the world? It depends how you define it.

So why is this the biggest computer programme in the world ever? Because it will computerise the medical records of the entire population of England – a population of 54 million people. And each record will consist of a bewildering collection of clinical and administrative data items. It will manage the day-to-day working processes of a million employees. It will manage the biggest, most dynamic, and fastest changing organisation in the West.

I think this makes it the biggest computer programme in the world ever. What do you think?

NPfIT is a rapidly changing programme and because of this, some of the detail and even nomenclature will have changed since going to press. However, the historical aspects are consistent and the fundamental NPfIT principles remain.

So what is this programme? How will it work? What lies behind this extravagant headstrong drive for new technology in healthcare? These are things that this book will explore.

Sean Brennan
February 2005

About the author

Sean Brennan has had a long career in the NHS starting in the Bolton hospitals in the early 70s, moving across the Pennines into Yorkshire in 1983 to take up the role of Chief Medical Laboratory Scientific Officer in Immunology at Huddersfield Royal Infirmary. He established a Medical Audit Unit at Huddersfield Royal Infirmary, ultimately becoming Information Manager with responsibility for the Resource Management, Medical Audit and IT staff.

In 1993, Sean was seconded to the Department of Health as a Clinical Audit Advisor. In 1996, he was appointed Project Manager for the NHS's national Electronic Patient Record Project in England, a position he held until 1999 when he had a dual role – split between the Health Department of the Scottish Office and the newly formed NHS Information Policy Unit in England.

In July 2000, Sean joined a computer supplier – Northgate Information Solutions (formerly MDIS) as Head of Healthcare Strategy, experiencing life in the commercial sector.

In 2002, Sean launched Clinical Matrix Limited, a network of consultants, engaged in strategy development, business cases, clinical change-management and general informatics projects for the NHS and commercial customers. Organising and facilitating interactive workshops with groups, large and small, is an area of particular interest and expertise with or without the interactive electronic voting keypads.

He is a part-time lecturer at Huddersfield University and at Derby University on health informatics and is regularly invited to speak at national and international conferences on health informatics issues.

Sean writes a monthly column for the *British Journal of Healthcare Computing & Information Management* called 'Down at the EPR Arms', a fictitious pub in Yorkshire where he reports on interesting conversations about health IT, www.eprarms.com.

Sean is married, lives in Huddersfield and has three daughters and a dog and can be contacted at sean.brennan@clinicalmatrix.com.

Acknowledgements

Because of the potential sensitivity of any book about the high profile National Programme for IT, there are many people who deserve my thanks but who would rather not receive them on this page. They know who they are and I am grateful for their advice and support.

I would like to thank Paul Brown, John Leach, Irving Mellor and Dr Bill Dodd who took the time and trouble to wade through this wordy manuscript and point out any factual errors for me and offer their feedback, and to Nettie de Glanville for her support and guidance.

I would especially like to express my gratitude to Dr John Ironmonger who provided great support during the re-writing stages.

Finally, as ever, to Kath, my wife, who has put up with my grumpiness as deadlines approached and to you, the reader, for buying the book.

Sean Brennan
February 2005

Dedicated to Mum and Dad,
Harry and Josephine Brennan.
May they rest in peace.

Chapter 1

Somewhere in the fog

The National Health Service is big. Very big. If you took every NHS employee and made them all hold hands in a chain, say a metre each apart, then the chain would stretch for almost 1400 kilometres. Conveniently, this is the exact distance by road from Land's End to John O'Groats (allowing for a few diversions along the way). Almost one in ten of the UK's working population depends upon the NHS for their income, either as an employee or as a supplier. No wonder, then, that any project that involves the whole NHS is necessarily going to be the biggest project in the country – if not the world. A project to repaint every NHS waiting room would probably be the biggest interior decoration project in history. Today, for example, one quarter of a million people will receive some NHS help in their homes.[1] If you are reading this on an average working day, then over one and a quarter million Britons will be seen by an NHS doctor today. That is a crowd that would fill out every seat at Manchester United 18 times over. 160 000 of those (or nearly two and a half Old Traffords) will be seen today during a hospital outpatient visit. Nearly 1500 babies will be born today, delivered by NHS midwives and doctors; hospital laboratories will report on the results of around five million tests, around 200 people will have hip replacement operations, and the global pharmaceutical industry can look forward to dispensing around one and a quarter million NHS prescriptions. Can you hear an ambulance siren? There will be over 7000 emergency ambulance trips today. And it's a typical day.

Yes, a typical day. But more things will happen today in the NHS than we might care to think about. The NHS will spend around £170 million of taxpayers' money today[2] – that works out to a little under £2000 every second. Surprisingly, around £10 million today will be spent settling litigation claims, which the National Audit Office[3] estimates as costing about £3.9 billion a year. Why are people suing the NHS? According to Dr Foster, a medical research firm (www.drfoster.co.uk), 110 people will die in NHS care today because of 'adverse events'. Other people put this number higher. The Office of Health Economics calculates about 173 deaths. Today. In NHS care. Effectively these people will have been killed accidentally because of mistakes in their treatment. That might be one reason why the litigation claims are so high. Can you imagine if the Post Office was accidentally to kill 173 people every day? Or the railways? We are surprisingly tolerant of this death rate, because we know in our hearts that the NHS is a benign organisation, doing its best to help us, not trying actively to kill us. But should we be so tolerant where these adverse events are due to poor management, inefficient processes, negligence, and easily avoidable human errors?

Thankfully not every 'adverse event' kills the patient. Today about 1230 patients will suffer one of these adverse events.[4] About 270 of these will fall victim to an infection today that they have contracted in hospital. That is quite an adverse event, and if you are a patient in an NHS hospital it may be little comfort to know that you have around a 9% chance of contracting such a bug. Around two to three people will die today in the NHS from one of the worst of these – an MRSA infection. MRSA is an acronym for methycillin-resistant *Staphylococcus aureus*. It is an infection almost exclusively contracted by patients in hospital, and the most common cause of infection is bad hygiene. Treating patients with MRSA infections will cost the NHS about £2.8 million today, and again tomorrow, and again the next day. Infection isn't the only adverse event that will impact patients in NHS care today, even though this is often the one that the newspapers seem most concerned with. It will cost the NHS £1.3 million today, and every day, just to treat patients for the effects of mistakes in prescribing.

So computerising the NHS is a logistical challenge as well as a technical one. It is a challenge of scale. Like the electrification of the Soviet Union, there is no way to do this on a small scale; and like the building of the Channel Tunnel, there isn't much point in only going half way. So big is this project, that even to people closely involved in it, the whole task can seem like a city enveloped in a fog. Like pedestrians in the fog, you can see the buildings around you reasonably clearly, but there is no single point which will give you a clear view of the whole city. Even if you climb a tall building for an aerial view, all you can see is a whole lot of fog.

To start with, the National Programme for IT (or 'NPfIT' as we must learn to call it) is only concerned with the NHS in England. It does not extend to Scotland, Wales, or Northern Ireland. In due course those regions may embark on programmes of their own. For now they are firmly outside NPfIT. Secondly, the National Programme is not, as it turns out, a single programme. The press often talks about 'a new computer system for the NHS', rather creating the impression of a single gigantic computer. In fact, eight separate programmes combine to make up the NPfIT. They are:

1 One NASP (National Application Service Provider) contract to provide the 'National Data Spine' – destined to become the biggest computer database in world history.
2 A New National Network (N3) – a broadband network to support all the applications and to connect GPs, hospitals and other health and social care providers across the country.
3 One project for Electronic Appointment Booking (eB) (now called 'Choose and Book').
4 Five Local Service Provider (LSP) 'cluster-wide' contracts to provide a NHS Care Records Service (NHS-CRS) at a local level – in the North West and West Midlands, in the North East and Yorkshire, in the East of England and East Midlands, in London, and in 'the South'.

Altogether this will amount to a lot more than 'a new computer system'. Ultimately there will be several hundred computer systems. But the key thing is that they will all be connected. And that, for the NHS, will be a wholly new event, as we shall see.

It appears that the first objective of NPfIT is to computerise patient records. That means that your record of encounters with the NHS, all your appointments and medications, all your doctor's notes and diagnoses, your test results and your X-rays, and countless other bits of information collected about you, as a patient, will be held on a computer. But that record won't create itself. So either the NHS

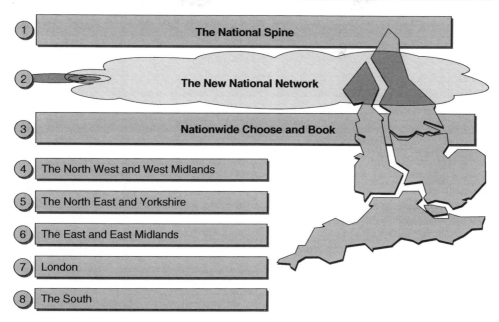

Figure 1.1 The National Programme for IT

will have to provide an army of data-input staff to type all that information into your electronic record, along with the systems to support all that activity, or else they have to create a way where the information is collected as part of the process of care. Here in a nutshell is the information challenge for the NHS. To provide you and me with a computerised patient record it won't be enough just to build a huge database and expect it to fill up with data. The NHS will need to introduce a system that will provide clinical support (which means helping care givers to do their job), and administrative support (which means helping administrators to do their jobs). This is the second objective of NPfIT. But it is so closely linked to the first objective that the two are hard to disentangle. Without providing tools to help the people who work in the health service, you won't get the electronic record that will help them to treat you properly.

The programme is intended to make use of technology to support the core objectives of the NHS. It is expected to deliver an improvement in the ability of clinicians (doctors and nurses) to track case notes (until the paper record becomes redundant), order tests and view the test results online, prescribe drugs and record and view other essential clinical information. It is also expected to provide a real-time view of a patient's status in the system, helping to reduce waiting times and improve clinical outcomes. Eventually it will offer NHS staff some streamlining of prescription ordering and appointment booking, and ultimately it will ensure that all healthcare organisations and all care settings from the doctor's surgery to hospitals, paramedics and social services have a single view of the patient, enabling more accurate diagnosis.

It is the boldest vision that any government has ever taken with respect to computing – and it comes against a historical background of high-profile failures in big government computer projects. So why is it happening? Have governments not learned anything from the disasters of the 1990s? And why is it costing so much and taking so long to deliver?

The answers, as you might expect, are complex, and hard to unravel. But one reason really stands out. Governments in Britain rise and fall upon their ability to manage a successful NHS. Every General Election brings a daily welter of statistics on waiting lists and outcomes, on the number of new nurses versus the number of administrators, on the number of ward closures, on the costs of dentistry and eye tests and prescription charges, on the prospects of contracting MRSA, on the hours worked by junior doctors, on nurses' salaries, and of your chances of surviving a heart attack in England compared with, say, France. Anecdotal stories of patients left on trolleys, of misdiagnoses, of errors and delays – these hog the tabloid headlines and drive the political agenda of every major party. The NHS can – and does – determine who wins and who loses where national politics is concerned. And yet there is a dreadful dilemma at the heart of all this, facing every occupant of Number 10. The costs and demands of healthcare are growing faster than the ability of the exchequer to pay for it all. The cold equations of healthcare have convinced even the most computer-sceptic parliamentarians that we can never find and recruit the number of nurses and doctors we need as demand grows – that even if we raid the medical schools and nursing colleges of Eastern Europe and Oceania in search of new recruits (as we have been doing) we cannot do this indefinitely. We need to do something else. We need to modernise the service. And that is going to take some serious IT.

In one of the meeting rooms of 10 Downing Street in February 2002 a routine meeting took place. It was a seminar where a clutch of very senior people would discuss the problems of the NHS, and try to explore ways to modernise the service. Round the table were Alan Milburn, the Secretary of State for Health, senior figures from the Department of Health and the Treasury and two IT companies. One of those companies was Microsoft. Whatever was said at that meeting, it has now become part of NHS history. A decision appears to have been taken that would start a train of events that would gather momentum in the weeks and months to come, until it became an unstoppable, invincible force. This decision was that a serious programme was needed to introduce information technology into the NHS in England. Previous IT initiatives, and there have been many (as we shall see), were dismissed as having been ineffective and insufficient. The NHS was not an IT organisation, yet it was expected to procure, operate and maintain thousands of computer systems. This was hardly the core business of a health service. One of the Downing Street decisions was, it appears, to outsource the huge computing responsibilities of the NHS to some very big companies, companies who should be able to bring massive expertise to the problem, who should be able to mobilise to build, deliver and support systems for almost a million users.

Who have been the key players in this unfolding drama? The Prime Minister, Tony Blair, of course; a decision of this magnitude can only have been made with his explicit support. The Health Secretary must have been persuaded that this would be a wise allocation of funds. The Chancellor, Gordon Brown, would have to have been close to the decision. Even though the price under discussion was 'only' around £2 billion at that time, it is unlikely that a decision to spend even this amount could have escaped his closest scrutiny. A man who appeared early on the scene was Professor Sir John Pattison. His job title at this point was seemingly innocuous. He was Director of Research at the Department of Health. His title belied his influence. From the start it seemed that it was Sir John's vision that was driving the programme in its early stages, and his judgement that was persuading the Whitehall mandarins. On 6 October 2002 a new figure appeared on the scene, recruited by Sir John. It was this man who was to become so closely associated with the programme that for much of the next two years this seemed like a personal campaign. His appointment was not without controversy. Joining from city consultants Deloittes, he became at once the highest paid civil servant in Britain on a reported salary of £250 000 a year. He came with a huge experience of public sector projects, with a famous no-nonsense approach. It was an early indication of the importance that Downing Street attached to the project. At the time of writing he is still Director General of NHS IT. His name is Richard Granger.

Among the barbs that were aimed at Granger in the early months of NPfIT was the accusation that there was no one at the heart of the programme who was seen to represent the doctors. This was resolved in January 2003 when Granger was joined by an obstetrician, Professor Aidan Halligan, formerly Deputy Chief Medical Officer, Director of Clinical Governance and Head of the Clinical Governance Support Team (CGST) for the National Health Service (NHS) in the United Kingdom. Professor Aidan Halligan, an Irishman, took up a position to join Richard Granger as joint Senior Reporting Officers for the programme, a post where he remained influential until his departure to become Chief Executive of the Irish Health Service in September 2004 – a post he subsequently did not take up.

How much is the National Programme going to cost?

We will probably never know. You may have seen the programme reported as a £2 billion project – or maybe as a £6 billion project – or maybe even more. It all depends on what we are counting – and for how long (and for purists, we seem to have finally settled on the American billion – or one thousand million). The first headline figure for NPfIT was £2.3 billion. This was the figure announced by Richard Granger, the Director General of NHS IT, in January 2003. The £6 billion number is also easy to understand. It represents the lifetime value of the contracts actually awarded – where each contract will run until 2013. These are:

Table 1.1

For what?	Awarded to?	Worth how much?
North East cluster	Accenture	£1,099,000,000
London cluster	BT (Capital Alliance)	£996,000,000
East & EM cluster	Accenture	£934,000,000
NW & WM cluster	CSC Alliance	£973,000,000
Southern cluster	Fujitsu Alliance	£896,000,000
The National Spine	BT	£620,000,000
Choose and Book	SchlumbergerSema (Now Atos Origin)	£64,500,000
New National Network	BT	£530,000,000
Totals		£6,112,500,000

But of course, there are costs that are not included in this total. In November 2004 the NHS struck a new three-year software licensing agreement with Microsoft, for example, for which it will pay a reported £500 million. There will be networking, infrastructure and devices at every site, which are not included in the contracts shown above. There are central management costs of NPfIT and the NHSIA. A £37 million, three-year contract was awarded in 2003 to consultants Kellogg Brown and Root to oversee the project planning, procurement support and implementation of the National IT Programme. The full value of this contract over 10 years could be worth up to £117 million. And then, of course, there are all the NHS employees who will be engaged full-time (or part-time) on the project between the time when the programme started – say in January 2003 – and when it finally comes to an end in 2013. At the very least this will add another £1 billion to the total. Add to all this the expectations of growth and new service additions by the existing service providers, termination costs for switching off legacy systems early, power, consumables, overheads, and cost overruns.

In October 2004 *Computer Weekly* ran a story that was quickly picked up by the national press and media forecasting that the total bill would fall around £18.6 billion and could rise to £31 billion. A figure of £40 billion was soon being discussed in the press. These figures were quickly dismissed as speculation by the health minister, John Hutton, who has responsibility for the National Programme. 'There is no evidence whatsoever that that this will be the cost of implementing the National Programme for IT,' he told Today programme listeners on BBC Radio 4. Hutton said instead that the £1 billion a year currently spent by the NHS on maintaining a 'hotchpotch' of 5000 separate systems should cover the costs of implementation. The figures appear to have originated from estimates drawn up by Department of Health officials and leaked to *Computer Weekly*. However, even pessimistic insiders would probably agree that they look unrealistically high.

A spokesman from the Department of Health was reported to have said, 'It is generally accepted in the IT industry that implementation costs are some 3–5 times the procurements and this is reflected in the business case that was made for the national programme.' That would explain the £18.6 billion figure.

But this kind of expenditure is exactly what was recommended by Derek Wanless in his review in 2002,[5] which suggested, although never explicitly stated, a doubling of investment in ICT, from 2% of total NHS budget to 4%.

Let us imagine that the current spend on computers and associated technology of a Strategic Health Authority may be, say, 1.4% of the authority's total budget. NPfIT will deliver an additional 1% centrally and the Strategic Health Authority will have to find an additional 1.6% (to make up the total ICT spend available to 4%), from local growth.

Whatever the final bill is, would anyone like to argue that the cost of NPfIT will not exceed, say £20 billion by the time it is all complete? As a service for England only, this would have cost the good people of England about £400 a head – or £40 each a year. Will it be £40 well spent? Let us find out.

Chapter 2

Modernising the service

When Gottlieb Daimler and Karl Benz built their first automobile in 1889. the vehicle they built looked more like a horse-drawn carriage than a motor car, and for decades to come, these 'horseless carriages' simply mimicked the design and appearance of the era that had come before. Daimler and Benz were bringing new technology to solve an old problem without realising that the technology itself was going to make such a fundamental change to transport that they could just about forget everything that had ever been developed to support horse-drawn transport, and start again with a clean sheet. Of course, it wasn't all due to a lack of imagination on their parts. They had the infrastructure of carriage-builders and wheelwrights and component makers and potholed roads to deal with, so maybe it was natural that their first instinct was to add their new technology to what was already there.

Sometimes history and infrastructure can become a very difficult thing to change. History is all around us – we are where we are because of what has gone before. Not just in healthcare. Railway lines in England are 4ft 8½ ins apart. But how did we settle on that curious dimension? It was because the first railway lines were built by the same people who built the pre-railway tramways, and that's the gauge they used. The people who built the tramways used this gauge because they used the same raw materials, jigs and tools that they used for building wagons, and wagons wheels were 4ft 8½ ins apart. If they weren't, then the wagon wheels would break on some of the old, long-distance roads which had well established ruts, 4ft 8½ ins apart. The original ruts were first made by the wheels of Roman war chariots, which were, you guessed it, 4ft 8½ ins apart. And so it is, in the twenty-first century, that the width of our railway carriages carries a genetic blueprint from Imperial Rome. If practices and processes can become as ingrained and as hard to shift as that, then we can start to see why an organisation like the NHS can be so difficult to change.

Consider the cycle of events that often happens when an organisation introduces IT. They start by computerising the existing processes, and then it soon dawns upon the organisation that maybe the old processes don't make a lot of sense anymore. Take an example from the airline industry. The process for buying an airline ticket used to be tortuous. You would visit your travel agent, who would do the booking for you. Lots of phone calls later, and after parting with your cash, your travel documents would arrive in the post as a sheaf of carbon paper slips that would be progressively torn off as you made your journey, exchanged for boarding cards that would be torn in half, and generally the process seemed designed to support a tier of airline staff whose main role appeared to be to check your documents. Even when computers arrived, the process barely seemed to change. The big sheaf of carbon paper slips in your ticket were now computer-printed instead of handwritten, and it did seem as if IT could do little more than save on ballpoint pens. No wonder air travel was expensive. Enter the budget airlines. You book on the Internet. No ticket, no boarding card, no frills. As a passenger your outcome is still the same – you reach your destination. Okay, you may not always arrive at the gleaming airport close to the city centre, but at an airfield with a Portakabin 30 miles out of town. But the price of your journey is half what it was when the old processes applied. The airlines now employ far fewer people per passenger, and so more people can travel. Airlines couldn't have done this without inventive and imaginative application of computer technology. So the lessons for the NHS are seductive. Could the NHS borrow something from the EasyJet experience? Could IT be used as a driver to change the processes from the familiar pattern of NHS behaviour to one where the patient outcomes were the same – or better – while the resources needed to get there were cut dramatically?

To understand how the NHS plans to computerise healthcare, let us assume to begin with that 'form will follow function'. In other words, the NHS already has a way of working, and so the technology delivered through the national programme will start by underpinning the work it already does. We know that simply supporting the existing workflows is not enough. But that is how it will probably need to start.

There is a simple formula to explain this phenomenon:

$$T + OS = EOS$$
$$\text{technology} + \text{old system} = \text{expensive old system}$$

In other words, we shouldn't just try to throw computers at the NHS without changing the way that the NHS works. New technology brings real opportunities to the NHS. Not just more shining computers, but better ways of working. Simply adding a layer of technology onto an old system of working will result in an expensive old system and an opportunity to improve will have been lost.

Having said all that, we have to start somewhere. So in assessing the opportunities for change, let us understand the way the NHS currently works and identify how technology could support its evolution.

If your only contact with the NHS to date has been as a patient, the following section might open your eyes to the vast numbers of people and services involved in delivering health and social care. The organisational structure is complex and constantly changing. That makes it all a real challenge.

The following scenarios are not clinically accurate, nor are they intended as criticism aimed at any of the hard-working people in the NHS. As Michael Crichton stated in the author's note to the republication of his 1969 book *Five Patients*:

> . . . the truth is that everyone works within the constraints of the present system – and it is the system itself that must be changed.

The patient's view

So let us consider the traditional patient journey today through the complex labyrinth of the NHS. Imagine you are Jimmy Rawthorpe. You are a 46-year-old builder, living and working in Huddersfield, and you feel ill. You telephone your

GP's receptionist who 'squeezes' you in a week on Tuesday. It's not her fault – the diary is chock-a-block.

You see the GP, who might either diagnose your problem and treat you, or send you for a battery of tests to help him diagnose, and then treat you. He examines you, and writes some forms for blood tests. 'Come back in a week for the results of the tests,' he might say.

So you do. He tears open an envelope and looks at some results from the laboratory. He sucks on a thoughtful tooth, and says nothing. At this point, if he is worried, he may refer you to a specialist at a local hospital.

You then wait for the specialist to send you an outpatient appointment. You receive a letter two weeks later advising you that an appointment has been made for four months on Wednesday.

You eventually attend the outpatient clinic and the specialist decides to do a battery of lab investigations (ignoring those previously done by the GP), again not his fault – not all the lab work requested by the GP is in the notes and the referral letter only gave a summary of those requested by the GP. He also requests some X-rays and makes an appointment for you to reattend in four weeks.

The specialist then reviews your results during your next outpatient appointment. Yes, during! It is often at this point, i.e. when you are sat there glumly in front of him, having waited four months, six weeks and 86 minutes, that he realises some of the test results haven't come back. He quickly scans the referral letter to remind him of the case, and his own notes (if he's seen you before), for what was planned. If you're lucky, he has all the results and he decides you need to be admitted for further investigations including an investigative operation in six weeks' time. In your case, some of the lab tests hadn't been done. So you have to reattend outpatients in another two weeks and then wait six weeks for your inpatient episode.

The six weeks drag by slowly and with each passing day your nervousness about your impending operation increases. Don't eat anything from the night before. Don't drink anything in the morning except 'sips' of water. Attend the Admissions office on the main ground floor. Bleary-eyed and nervous, you find somewhere to park very easily. That makes a change. Mind you, at 7 o'clock in the morning there are only burglars and milkmen about.

You sit fidgeting outside the admissions office and a clerk eventually arrives with a trolleyload of thick paper notes. She calls out your name and sits you next to an old-fashioned, steam-driven computer while she checks your name and age and religion and address. She then points you to the lifts and tells you to go to the third floor and ring the bell for Ward 34.

You do all this obediently. You are on foreign turf and completely subservient and worried. Your life is now firmly in their hands. On the ward you are taken to a bed, told to change into your pyjamas (which you had previously gone out and bought specially), and you wait. The ward is a hive of activity with all sorts of uniforms coming in, doing tasks, leaving. No one speaks to you.

Your named nurse is Britney a sign above your bed tells you. If only! A nurse (Britney you assume) comes and clerks you in. Checks your name, your age, your address, your religion. She goes through the procedure with you. You will have to wait on the bed till they take you down to theatre. When? 'Can't tell you that. It may be after lunch.' What? 'Oh no – you can't have any lunch. Nothing by mouth till after the op.'

So let's recap. How long has it been?

- A week and a half waiting for your GP appointment.
- A further week waiting for lab tests.
- Two weeks waiting for an outpatient appointment letter telling you of a date for the outpatient appointment.
- Four months waiting for outpatient clinic appointment.
- Four weeks waiting for results of tests before repeat outpatient appointment.
- Another two weeks while they repeat the tests that didn't end up in your notes or didn't get done in the first place.
- Six weeks to be admitted.

And the cost. You have to take a day off work for each appointment. That's one for the GP. Three for outpatients. At least the inpatient episode is classed as sick leave. A day off for the post-op outpatient check. That's nearly a week's wages. And a week's holiday gone.

Luckily for you, at least the right specialist was chosen for your problem, 'cos if not, you'd have to go through that whole cycle again!

But it's no one's fault. It's the way it works. Remember Michael Crichton: '. . . the truth is that everyone works within the constraints of the present system – and it is the system itself that must be changed'.

Experience Jimmy's episode: become Jimmy for a while.

An important looking group of people is heading down the ward, from bed to bed, heading your way. Led by a chap in a suit . . . he's the one you saw in outpatients. Mr Bob something or other. He's standing at the end of the beds, reviewing the paper notes of the patient next door. You're next. He's surrounded by an assortment of uniforms. A tired junior doctor struggling to keep awake after a bad night on call. Nurses, pharmacist, other uniforms you don't recognise. Your turn. Be calm. Be cool.

The gang approach and the suit holds out his hand to the staff nurse for the paper notes. 'Right,' he says, quickly flicking through the paper, knowing exactly where everything he needs is. To the referral letter. Flick to his outpatient notes. Flick to the lab results. 'I will be operating on you this afternoon. I am just going to see what we can find down there' – gently palpating your stomach – 'and then I'll come and see you after the operation. Any questions?'

'Millions,' you think, but you say, 'None spring to mind thanks.'

You are slightly overawed and underdressed and regret buying the 'cool' Homer Simpson jim-jams with an obese Homer stood holding a beer can in one hand and chicken leg in the other with 'Simply Irresistible' boldly printed under the swollen, jaundiced character of Homer. It seemed like a good idea when you were choosing them in Asda yesterday. Not a pyjama person, you were making a statement. Now you just feel a prat.

'No questions,' you hear yourself saying and with that they move on to the next bed with one of the nurses noticing the pyjamas and giving you a strange look.

So you're lying on the bed and have been since eight this morning. It's now two in the afternoon and no one can tell you when you will be going to theatre. 'Very soon now' was all they would say, and that was an hour ago. Oh what's this? Activity? A chap in a white coat over green theatre scrubs is heading your way with your fat paper notes. 'Can I just check your details?' he asks politely. 'Name, date of birth? Right. I am Dr Singh, your anaesthetist. I will be looking after you during the operation. I just need to ask you some questions.'

Here we go again, you think. I've already been through all this 10 times over. No – you've no history of heart disease. No you don't smoke. 'I will be back to give you some medicine to make you drowsy, in about an hour. OK?' 'OK,' you say. Let's get on with it.

You are back alone on your bed with a flutter of trepidation in your stomach. 'I wonder what they will do to me?' you think. 'What will they find? Will it hurt? Will I die under anaesthetic?' Control the panic. Count to 10.

'Count down from 10 for me,' the anaesthetist says as he starts injecting a drug into a butterfly-type needly-thing they've taped to your forearm. You are now in the cold operating theatre – in a small room next to the one where a gaggle of assorted scrub suits are loitering around a big stainless steel table. It is an alien environment and you are totally and completely at their mercy. Whatever they want to do to you they can do.

The anaesthetist has been true to his word and came back to your bed within an hour and gave you some syrupy medicine which made you less stressed and fearful. He went away and eventually a porter and a nurse came to put you on a trolley. You saw the hospital from a new angle – the ceilings of the ward, the corridor, the lift, counting the fluorescent tube lights on the ceiling as they flashed by, slowing while the corridor ended with the big flappy plastic doors of what you presumed to be the operating theatre. You hear strange mechanical noises and are aware of a lot of people being very busy and knowing what they are doing.

You are wheeled into a very small room with shelves and cupboards and nurses and Dr Singh. So much activity and you are at the centre of it. 'Ten, nine, eight.' You'll show them.

You'll get down to one if it's the last thing . . .

Strange gassy noises wake you. Long, drawn-out breathy sounds. It's coming from . . . it's coming from you! You have a gas mask air-tube thing on your nose and you are back on your bed. You're alive. Praise the Lord. Whatever has happened, you are still here. Whatever the pain, you are still breathing. You wonder what they found. Is it good news? Is it bad? Whatever. You are still in the land of the living.

A smaller gang approach your bed but this time the suit man is wearing his green theatre garb.

'Right. Erhmm,' looking at your paper notes, 'Mr Rawthorpe. I've had a look inside you and found some inflammation in there which I will control with some drugs. I will keep you in for another day and you could go home on Wednesday. Any questions?'

Again, you hear yourself saying no.

The 'one day' eventually turned into five as you reacted to some of the drugs they gave you, which resulted in a nasty rash, which in turn needed some more drugs and cream.

All in all, it's been a miserable time and you couldn't wait to get home, which you did – exactly one week after you were first admitted.

You were given an outpatient appointment for eight weeks after discharge, which you went to. Another day off work; another struggle finding a place to park.

And to cap it all, you didn't see Surgeon Bob in outpatients. You saw a young lad fresh from school who didn't know you from Adam.

He read through the notes, had a quick palpate, asked you if you'd had any problems, and then discharged you. What a waste of a day's annual leave.

Still, the pain's gone and it's not their fault. It's nobody's fault really, is it?

But there's got to be a better way.

The GP's view

Busy, busy, busy. Waiting room full again of sniffling people and crying babies. A patient every seven and a half minutes. Surgery lasts two hours. Ten minutes allocated per appointment. That's 12 patients per surgery. That's a laugh. I regularly have 15 every surgery. But I still have to give them time. So I am always chasing my tail. The patients wait. The patients are grumpy. I am stressed, harassed. And yet the next one to walk through my door could have something seriously wrong with them. Or they may not.

I read the paper notes of the patient due in next. Not much in these notes. He's not a malingerer. No ongoing current problem. No idea why he's coming to see me. Better let him in now.

Talk to patient. Abdominal pain. Examine him. Look for obvious causes. Mmmm. Could be anything. Better do some tests and see him again in a week. Put prescription pad away. Can't prescribe anything yet. Write some laboratory request forms.

A week later

Surgery full of sniffling folk and crying babies. Next patient. Look at the paper notes. Ah this chap came to see me a week ago. I sent for some tests. Mmmm. Some slight elevation of white cell count. Amylase is raised.

Now then. He's more tender now than he was. Not sure what this is. Better refer him to the specialist. But which one? Erhm – well, it's not gynaecological. It's not bone (orthopaedic). It's not the tube man (urological) – too high up. Not skin (dermatological) – too deep. I'll refer him to a surgeon. I'll send him to Bob. This is his general area and he's a good mate. Playing cricket with him against the private hospital soon. Must go and have a drink with him sometime. I'll write a referral letter, telling him what I've found and the results of the tests I've requested.

'You will hear from the specialist soon who will give you an outpatient appointment. Goodbye.'

Now, who's next? Just another 10 to see before I go out on my rounds.

Four months later

Four months later and I'm going through my post before doing my visits. Letters from drug companies, various hospital lab reports, outpatient letters, A&E letters, discharge letters. Oh, lots today. All have to be seen and then filed in the patient's notes. I wish we could have these electronically – I could just put them into the patients' electronic records.

'I wish we could have these electronically Julie,' I say to the receptionist. 'It would save you having to type them into the computer, wouldn't it.'

'Wouldn't it just,' she said, opening an envelope 'Oh – here's another. An outpatient letter about Jimmy Rawthorpe.'

'Who? Ah yes – abdo pain. That was months ago. Does it say much?'

'Nope – they're doing more tests.'

'Oh, just stick it in his files. I'm going out on my rounds now, just phone me if anything urgent crops up.' And with that I get into my battered but serviceable Discovery.

Six weeks later

I get another letter telling me that the abdo pain is still there and the lab results are inconclusive and that Jimmy Rawthorpe needs to be admitted to hospital for a laparotomy. Jimmy Rawthorpe. That was ages ago. Can't remember him what he had wrong with . . . oh yes, Jimmy. Abdo pain. Not seen him since that first appointment. Wonder how he's doing?

Two months later . . .

'Morning Julie,' I say with a degree of optimism. A new week and all is good. Not for long. They've run out of teabags again and the coffee in front of you is decaff. Not what you need first thing in the morning.

'Post!' says Julie, equally feeling the strain of the caffeine deficiency, as she unceremoniously drops a pile on the table.

I start to flick my way through them. No, I don't need a credit card. No, I don't have time to go to a lecture on 'Parasitic Infections in Africa', and I certainly don't need to subscribe to a new journal. I've not enough time to read the ones I currently get.

Ah, now, lab test results. Mmm, they don't mean a lot without digging out the paper records. I can't remember this case. Outpatient letters and discharge letters. Mmm . . . had one or two in hospital recently. Didn't know that. Oh, and they've been home now for several weeks too! Didn't know that either. Why doesn't anyone tell me these things?

Oh – Jimmy Rawthorpe. Yes, went to see his mum yesterday. She said that Jimmy's been in hospital. It's bad when you hear it from the patient's relatives isn't it?

So what did they find? Mmm. Oh dear! Problems. A rash. A week ! He was in a week! Oh dear. Ah well, at least he's sorted now. Must make a note about his drug sensitivity – do it later. Must get some teabags first, and then start on this week's patients . . .

Two months later still . . .

'Good morning, Doctor,' says Julie with a smile. Now that's a first! Wonder what she's been up to? Perhaps with a smile like that she shouldn't be on the front desk.

'Morning Julie. Another day, another dollar.'

'Here's your post today. Just some outpatient letters so far,' she says as she hands me a small pile of paper.

I shuffle through them, coming across one for Jimmy Rawthorpe. A brief note saying . . . Mmmm everything is OK, settled down to treatment, discharged back into the GP's care. I make a note to have the patient come in and see me. If I have to wait for him to contact me, it could be ages.

Did he really have to go all the way back to hospital for his post-op check? Losing a day's wages, and that parking! Why couldn't I have done that check for them? It's not as if the surgeon himself did it. It was probably one of his young juniors.

Anyway, I've enough to do without adding fresh work, and I certainly haven't time to start changing the way I work. It's easier just to keep battling on.

But there's got to be a better way.

The specialist's view

Just finished my operating theatre list. Time to do a quick ward round before I go to the outpatient clinic. But first let's catch up with my paperwork. 'Any new referrals Gladys?' I ask my secretary.

She's very organised and gives me a folder with a mixed assortment of letters from GPs of varying quality.

> Dear Mr W,
>
> I am apparently referring this patient to you! Unfortunately I can't find any records as to why, but I'm sure you will find out!
>
> Regards

They're not all that bad. Here's a good one.

> Dear Bob,
>
> Re James Rawthorpe
>
> This patient came to me complaining of abdominal tenderness which is tender to the touch. Not appendix.
>
> Lab work done shows elevated WCC and Amylase but everything else normal.
>
> I would be grateful if you could see him and let me know your opinion.
>
> Kind regards and see you at the cricket match next Sunday.
>
> Peter

Send him an appointment, Gladys – next available. Right, I'm just going on the wards and then clinic till five. Leave all letters for signing and I'll do them later.

Four weeks later . . .

Just finished my operating theatre list. Time to do a quick ward round before I go to the outpatient clinic. But first, let's catch up with my paperwork.

'Any new referrals Gladys?' I ask my secretary, who gives me a folder with a mixed assortment of letters from GPs of varying quality.

Having sorted them, I go to my ward round. Had a number of unexpected admissions overnight so I get delayed and eventually arrive at the clinic an hour late. The clinic waiting room is really crowded today, with people standing. I see the nurse asking the patients to move from one chair to another. 'Mrs Jones, can you sit over here please. Mr Finney, over here.' It keeps the patients moving, they think they are moving through the system. But actually, they're not. Once they've sat on all chairs, they're sent home! Not really – anyway, at least it prevents DVTs. I grab my trolley of notes and enter my room.

Right, first patient. I flick through the heavy notes, scanning the referral letter and flick through existing current notes. None. This is a new patient. Reasonable referral letter.

Dear Bob,

Re James Rawthorpe

This patient came to me complaining of abdominal tenderness which is tender to the touch. Not appendix.

Lab work done shows elevated WCC and Amylase but everything else normal.

I would be grateful if you could see him and let me know your opinion.

Kind regards and see you at the cricket match next Sunday.

Peter

We lost that game again – against the private hospital. Still, the food was good. Right; better see him. What time was his appointment? Oh – 2 o'clock. Time now: 3:26. Ooops. 'Mr Rawthorpe please,' I ask the nurse.

The patient comes in. Looks a bit frustrated that he's been waiting. Probably thinks I've been playing golf or doing private work. Doesn't realise I've been on the go since 6:30 this morning after a rushed cup of tea, and won't get home till after eight tonight. I thought it was supposed to be the junior doctors that got this abused.

'OK Mr Rawthorpe. What's your problem?'

While the patient gives me the details I start prodding and poking, palpating and touching. All the while I am listening and 'mmmming' and 'Fine, OK'. What could it be? I allow a clinical algorithm to go through my mind. Let's exclude X and Y. If there's no pain here then it's not Z. That narrows it down a bit. But it could still be any number of conditions. Let's have a look at the lab work. Uh-oh – I've only got the GP's summary of what he's done. White cells raised. High serum Amylase. Everything else is normal. Yes but what other tests did he do, and how normal were they? I need to have more lab work and perhaps an X-ray.

'OK. Put your shirt back on now. I need some more work doing on you. I want you to have some blood tests.'

'But I've already had blood tests.'

'Yes but I need some more. And an X-ray. So see the receptionist on the way out and come and see me again in, say, four weeks. OK?'

The patient reluctantly takes the lab request forms. Obviously he was hoping for a quick resolution. But how can I sort this out without the information? I suppose he's worried he has to take another day off work to come and see me. And the car parking. Yes it is a pain being a patient.

Ah well. 'Next patient nurse.'

Another grumpy individual comes in looking like thunder . . .

Four weeks later . . .

Just finished my operating theatre list. Some tricky ones today. One overran by 40 minutes. That caused a knock-on effect throughout the whole of theatres. 'Why can't you tell us when I am going down to theatre?' they ask while sitting, gowned-up on their ward bed. 'Well, actually its 'cos I haven't a bloody clue,' I would love to say.

Time to do a quick ward round before I go to the outpatient clinic. But first, let's catch up with my paperwork.

'Any new referrals, Gladys?' I ask my secretary, who gives me a folder with a mixed assortment of letters from GPs of varying quality – again. Another Groundhog Day. 'Oh OK. I'll do those later,' I say when Gladys asks if I've done the discharge letters yet which are piling up on my desk.

Having sorted them, I go to my ward round. I spend a bit of time with those I've just operated on, especially the difficult case, currently on ICU. They've put one of my patients right at the other end of the hospital, on a gynaecology ward no less. I nearly forgot. Damn – I'm going to be late for clinic again. And I've got my clinical audit meeting to get ready for, and a Trust Board meeting about some computer project. Hah. Where will I find the time for all that?

Clinic is very busy today again. Queuing at the desk. Standing room only. I dodge quickly past the angry stares. I would love to stop and tell them what kind of a day I've had. But no time. Straight in.

First patient. Where are the notes? Ah here they are. Flicking through the notes I read my last clinic notes first. Flick back to the referral letter. Flick back to my notes. Oh yes I remember. Not enough information. Requested lab tests. X-rays. Flick to the radiologist's report. Mmmm, nothing specific. Lab work. Flick down the coloured report forms. Where's the Biochemistry? There's one report there but the serum 'rhubarb' is missing. Oh bugger. Bugger. Bugger. I'm still as much in the dark. I need that test result.

'Nurse. Can you phone Biochem and chase this result up please?' I'll take the next patient while we are waiting.

Good, this one's routine. Flick through the notes. Give a quick check. No complications. Surgery went well. Lab work OK. Good. Finished.

I suppose the patient is wondering why a 90-minute wait for a three-minute assessment has cost him a day's wages. I bet he wonders why the GP couldn't have done that for me. Or a specialist nurse. But he's my patient. I am accountable. I have to make sure I am sending him out into the world completely OK. 'You're completely OK, Mr Jones. I will write to your GP but I don't have to see you again.'

The nurse comes in. Pretty little thing she is.

'What – they haven't done the tests? Why not? They never received it? Oh bugger. Bring him in.'

I'll examine him anyway and get some more tests done. 'Mr Rawthorpe. I'm sorry but I need these tests before I can be sure what's wrong with you. I will have to ask you to have some more tests. Go to the lab and come and see me again in two weeks' time. OK?'

If looks could kill.

'Next patient please, nurse.' Cor! I'm starving. Not eaten today again. Have to call in at the WRVS shop when I've done here.

Two weeks later . . .

What a night! Called in at three o'clock for an emergency op which ended up in ICU. Must have a word with the family today. Not much hope. Will have to ask them about switching off the life support. What a job. Oh, and I mustn't forget to ask them about donating their loved one's organs. What a time to hit them with that question.

Ah well, must rush down the corridor into Outpatients. At least I'm on time today! Mind you, I've not been home yet. Eyes prickly and feeling a bit grubby, I sit at my desk and pick up the first set of notes.

Jimmy . . . now what is this one about? Flicking through the notes, I remind myself of the story so far. Abdo pain. Mmm, lab tests – weren't all there, had to do them again. Ah here they are. Good. X-rays. Mmm. OK – I'd better get him in.

'Bring him in please, nurse,' I ask the staff nurse.

'Mr Rawthorpe. Good to see you. How's the tummy? Oh, the same? OK, I have the results of all tests now and I think we'd better bring you in for an operation. I need to have a look around you. No, it's not a big operation, but you will have a general anaesthetic and I will have to open up your tummy about there. Should be in and out within a couple of days. What? No, I don't know when that will be. You will get a letter. OK? Any questions? No? Good. Bye.'

And with that I pick up the next set of notes and flick through to remind myself of the next case.

'Next.'

Six weeks later . . .

Theatre day today. First, do a ward round. Oh, I wish they wouldn't split my patients up like this. These two here on Ward 34, and then three more patients at the other end of the hospital on Ward 10. I'll be doing some mileage today.

Let's see who I have on the list today: One gall bladder removal and laparotomy. The two colorectal jobbies and a haemorrhoid. And a working lunch first. Something about computerising the hospital. Probably so that management can keep their eye on me! Don't trust computers. I have enough trouble at home with it locking up. I don't need that at work too! Last thing I need is to have my ward round delayed while we 'Ctrl-Alt-Delete' to start it up again. And I hate typing. What will my juniors think of me and my two-fingered typing?

No, that's not for me. I'll steer well clear of that nonsense. If they want computers, they can jolly well do all the typing. I'm not going to change the way I work, and I don't want to look daft, do I ? Cor, I'm grumpy today aren't I!

OK, let's get started. 'Are we ready for the ward round?' I ask, gathering together my team, who assemble behind me hierarchically. It's nothing I've told them to do – it just happens. Once auto-arranged, we set off down the ward.

I stand at the end of the first bed, reviewing the paper notes of the newly-admitted patient for gallbladder removal. I tell them the usual: 'little keyhole job', should be home later today. No problems.

I walk on to the next bed accompanied by my army of assorted uniforms. Andrew Castle looks tired. These junior docs don't know they're born. In my day, I'd think nothing of working seven days and nights straight through with no sleep. They think nothing of it either! Junior doctors' hours! Rotas! Pah! All that extra work for me.

I hold out my hand to the staff nurse for the paper notes. 'Right', I say quickly flicking through the paper . . . referral letter. Flick to outpatient notes. Flick to lab results. 'I will be operating on you this afternoon. I am just going to have a look around, see what's going on down there,' gently palpating the patient's stomach, 'and then I'll come and see you after the operation. Any questions?'

The patient – erhm . . . Jimmy Rawthorpe – shrugs as if he's considering a multitude of questions and settles on 'None spring to mind, thanks'.

What hideous pyjamas he's got on. That's the Simpson character, isn't it? I wonder if he realises that he looks like a prat!

Ok, so on we go to the next ward. What a hike – almost a mile.

Eventually I return to my office where my secretary has all the new correspondence for me to read, and some she has just typed for me to sign.

Fast approaching lunch, I quickly scan-read the correspondence, making notes for my secretary to action. I sign the discharge letters I dictated last night. Yes, the patients have been discharged several weeks ago, but I can only do so much.

Done. And so to my working lunch. It had better be quick, my theatre list starts at one. Computers? Pah!

Scrub. Scrub. I wonder if Semmelweis is happy now? All this scrubbing. And yet we still have the odd MRSA infection problems. Well, it's not coming from these hands, that's for sure.

Here we go. This is what I like best – surgery. This is what it's all about. Let's hope it all goes smoothly today.

But it doesn't. It starts off badly with the 'little keyhole jobbie' turning into a major operation. The gall bladder was very fragile and swollen and I decided to dispense with the time- (and scar-) saving keyhole surgical procedure and opt for the open cholecystectomy. Once the patient was completely opened up, the removal of the offending swollen organ was relatively simple, but it had put me back in my list. I was now running late. Here we go again, chasing my tail.

While the patient is wheeled into recovery, I take the notes and a cup of coffee into the staff room and write my theatre letter.

A quick stretch, another scrub, and it's the next one. Flick through the notes to remind myself why the patient – erhm . . . Jimmy Rawthorpe – is here. Laparotomy. OK. Open him up, have a scoot round. Severe inflammation, no obvious cause, rinse. Antibiotic wash.

Done. Send him back.

Write letter.

Next!

Colorectal. Let's see if we can get to the bottom of this one! (The old ones are the best.)

Three hours later and still in my theatre greens, I visit each of my patients now back on their wards. Quick glance at my theatre notes and tell them reassuring things about their case. Back to the office to do some more letters, and then home.

Wonder what's on the telly tonight? I'm knackered.

Four weeks later . . .

'. . . And I'll just do the letters and I can be found on the golf course if needed urgently.'

Taking an armful of fat paper notes with me and a cup of coffee, I sit in the quiet office and slowly dictate the discharge letters for the last week or two. They've been piling up. Not had time. Getting to the last one, I began to imagine a nice quiet afternoon chasing a little ball around the grass with a stick.

'. . . And finally, a letter to Dr Peter Barnes, at Westbourne.

'Dear Peter, re Jimmy Rawthorpe. Thanks for referring this patient to me. As you know, I saw Jimmy in outpatients where I did some lab work which, whilst repeating your raised white cell count result and a high Amylase, was pretty inconclusive. I admitted him and performed a laparotomy on the . . . ' (now, when was it . . . flick flick . . . four weeks ago, that'd be . . .) '27th September.

'We found some inflammatory changes, but no obvious evidence of an acute problem.

'We put Jimmy on antibiotics, but he reacted to them. Has he ever experienced a penicillin allergy before? There's no mention in his notes or in your referral letter. As a result, we had to keep him in till his rash subsided. He was discharged on the 3rd October and is due in clinic in eight weeks' time.

'Kind regards

'Etc. etc.'

Have to be careful what you write in letters and notes these days. Patients actually see what's in there now! What's the world coming to?

'Gladys. I'm off now. Can you type these and I'll sign them first thing Monday morning. Bye!'

I shouldn't be seeing Jimmy again. My junior will do the post-op clinic check. It's only a routine series of questions. Don't know why we drag the poor patient all the way up here to hospital, to be honest. Still, I'm too busy to change the way we work.

But there's got to be a better way.

Wouldn't it be better if . . .

Perhaps there is a better way. Perhaps the extraordinary paper-chase and catalogue of delays that typifies Jimmy Rawthorpe's journey through the NHS could be swept away and replaced by something more dynamic. Jimmy's experience is a fictional one, but is so typical of the experience of every NHS patient who has ever been bounced between GP and specialist and placed on a seemingly interminable waiting list, that most of us can probably identify with it from some personal experience. Yet there is something ludicrously old-fashioned about the process, with its handwritten notes and missing results and oversights and errors and delays. It hearkens back to an era before we had technology to help cut though all this wasteful paper-jam. It has echoes of a centralised, bureaucratic, almost Orwellian system about it, with its apparent disregard for the patients or even for the staff who operate within it. And yet it is a process so deeply etched into the fabric and minds of the NHS that even the victims of the process resist attempts to change it.

But change it must. We talked earlier about the National Programme as if it was a fog, enveloping a city. It is hard to see the shape of the fog, but we can see things around us clearly. So in this book we are going to have to zoom in a lot and consider the detail before we can really explore the vision that the government has.

Let us imagine that vision – 10 years hence.

We'll start by zooming in through the fog, right into Edith Road in Huddersfield. We met a patient, James Rawthorpe, in the scenarios above – so now let's meet his mum. Hilda Rawthorpe is an old lady with some problems. Well, not that old. She's 74, and even though she has a bus pass she still stays pretty active. She walks every day to the shops, and only takes the bus to the library. She helps out at the primary school with domestic science, and does the flowers at church. She lives alone. Her husband John died over 20 years ago of a bad heart. Her children are grown up now, with children of their own. Hilda doesn't grumble. She still sees them quite regularly – well, as often as can be expected 'cos they've all got busy lives. Her youngest son, Jimmy, was quite ill some years ago. Spent time in hospital and things didn't go as well as they had hoped. Still, he's through that now.

She too has her problems. She has a difficult hip, and she's on a waiting list for a replacement. But she stays cheerful. Last Christmas her consultant told her she had diabetes. It's something to do with sugar in the blood, apparently. But according to Doctor Rose it helps to explain her aches and pains, why she was always thirsty and tired, and why she'd been losing weight. Now she's supposed to check her blood sugar every day by pricking her fingertip with a little pen. Actually it is something of a hassle. It doesn't hurt – well not much. But she's never got particularly good at doing it. On Monday, when Eastenders was on, a little reminder popped up in the corner on her television set. 'Please remember to test your blood sugar,' it said. 'Would you like to do the test now?'

Why does it always wait until the soaps begin before it reminds you? She waited until the documentary at nine o'clock, and then went out and found the testing kit. It read twelve point five. She punched the number out on her television remote control.

'Thank you for entering your test result' said the message. 'You entered a result of 12.5 mmol/l. This means your blood sugar is running a little high. What time was your last meal?'

Hilda thought about this. She had eaten a biscuit or two at eight o'clock, but did that really count? She hadn't actually eaten a meal this evening, not a proper cooked meal, but she felt that this was not what the television wanted to know. So she pressed the arrow buttons and chose 5.00 pm. That would do. It seemed to satisfy the TV. Now back to the documentary.

'You are running low on testing pens.' It's at it again. 'Press the red button if you would like to order a new set?'

Hilda pressed the red button hoping this was the last question. But there was more.

'We can deliver this to you at home, or if you like you can collect it from Boots in the High Street. Press red if you want us to deliver, and green if you would like to collect this yourself.'

Hilda pressed the red button. 'Thank you,' said the TV message. 'A new pack will be delivered to you at 27 Edith Road Huddersfield on Wednesday between 10.00 am and midday.'

She thought that was the end, but then a new message appeared. 'Dr Rose has suggested that you should come and see her if your blood sugar starts to rise beyond 12 mmol/l. Would you like to make an appointment now? Press the red button, or press green to make your appointment later.'

Hilda sighed. She pressed the green button. All this computer stuff was tiring.

But that was all on Monday. Now it was Thursday and she hadn't tested her blood again, even though the television reminded her every time she turned it on. She was tired. And her whole body ached. That mobile phone that Jimmy had bought for her kept beeping, but when she tried to answer there was no one on the other end. Jimmy knew how these things worked, but she couldn't work it out. The last time this happened Jimmy told her that this was a text message from the hospital. She slumped down in her armchair and tried to reach for the remote control. It was out of reach. The room seemed to be turning. She felt curiously dizzy.

At Ambulance control in Halifax, an alert began to flash on a computer screen. Zoe Kelsall was at her desk. An elderly patient was causing some concern. A monitor at her home had reported that she had stayed in her armchair overnight. She hadn't moved. The toilet had not been flushed. On its own that might have been enough to raise an alarm – but this patient was also diabetic and her blood sugar had not been tested for some days. Zoe checked the graph. Okay. For a month or so Hilda's blood sugar a couple of hours after a meal had been fairly steady at seven or under. But the graph showed it had been rising slowly. Zoe hit the mouse button.

As Ambulance Seven idled by the traffic lights in Huddersfield, a beep came from the onboard control screen. 'Edith Road,' thought George as he glanced at the on-screen map. Just a couple of streets away.

For Dr Nita Patel this was only her third day on A&E. It had been hard work, but not as harrowing as she had feared. Broken bones mainly, cuts and bruises.

She unzipped the case that carried her tablet PC – funny how this had become as important a tool in medicine as the stethoscope, she thought. There didn't seem much to it. Just like a laptop screen and a clever electronic pen that she could carry around with her. She was new enough to the technology to be apprehensive as she slipped her smartcard out of her top pocket, and slid it into the device. What if it wouldn't let her log on? With no keyboard in sight, she scribbled her PIN number onto the screen and a couple of seconds passed. Then the inevitable hourglass, and then a welcome screen. 'Welcome Dr Nita Patel' read the screen. She slung the device over her shoulder and started to walk off down the corridor. In this job there was no time to be indulgent with computers. These things were a tool for the job, nothing more. As she walked, however, she glanced at the screen. Sixteen e-mails! Already! She grimaced. Heaven knew when she would have time to read them all. The screen showed a schematic map of the A&E department. Little dots represented the patients – some in reception, some in examination rooms, some in X-ray. The dots changed colour from green to amber to red depending upon how long they had been waiting.

Before Nita swished open the curtains of the first examination room, she tapped her pen onto the dot that represented the patient waiting within. Up popped a new screen. 'Hilda Rawthorpe' read a bold line at the top, followed by Hilda's age and date of birth. Nita wasn't overfamiliar with this new computer system, but you didn't need to be an expert to read *this* screen. Hilda had triggered an automated alert when she fell into a diabetic coma last night. Ambulance staff had treated her and bought her in. A scrolling graph right there on Hilda's front screen showed her slowly rising blood tests. A note at the top also made Nita raise an eyebrow. Hilda was on a clinical pathway waiting for a hip replacement in the next few weeks. She clicked on the screen to send a note to Hilda's consultant. If there were complications caused by the diabetic episode, then he would want to know, it might cause a variation in the planned pathway of care. Otherwise, who knows, maybe the operation could be brought forward.

And so this is the vision of the future. Not science fiction but science fact.

The National Programme for IT is nothing less than an ambitious plan to leverage technology into the whole delivery process for healthcare, so that stories like Hilda Rawthorpe's stop being fiction and simply become commonplace; everyday stories about the NHS delivering better care for its millions of users. Every piece of this jigsaw already exists – perhaps not in Huddersfield, perhaps not for Hilda Rawthorpe, but none of this actually needs to be invented. It is here already. This is what technology can already do for healthcare.

Imagine what might have happened to Jimmy. Instead of visiting his GP he goes to one of the new NHS walk-in diagnosis and treatment centres. Before he even sees a doctor a triage nurse orders a routine profile of blood and urine tests and sends him for an abdominal X-ray. A nurse takes some blood and sticks a bar code label on the bottle and passes it through a window to the laboratory. The lab technician simply pops the bottle into an analyser machine. The bar code on the bottle will tell the analyser who the sample belongs to, and what tests to do, and the results will go straight back to the computer. When Jimmy sees the specialist 40 minutes later, the results of those tests and the image from the X-ray are already there on the consultant's tablet computer. Labs are so fast these days. The specialist checks the theatre schedule. 'I'm putting you in for a small operation this afternoon,' he says. 'The nurse will take you to the day ward.' The computer shows that Jimmy is allergic to penicillin. That's okay. It won't let anyone prescribe it. Jimmy should be back home tonight.

Tonight? Isn't this a process that took several months back in 2004? Could it really happen in less than a day?

Remember the experience of the budget airlines. Technology isn't about supporting the old processes. It is about introducing new ones. And this is what this book is about.

Chapter 3

How is the NHS organised?

Before we consider how the NHS is to introduce computers across its entirety, it would be helpful to understand its complex structure and interrelationships, coupled to its constantly changing shape.

The NHS has been in a process of almost continuous reorganisation since its inception in 1948. Whole tiers of organisational structure have disappeared in that time to leave what is now a relatively slim organisation. Not that you might think so, however, when you hear the vitriol heaped by politicians and tabloid papers onto NHS managers. But then accusing the NHS of spending too much money on managers and not enough on doctors and nurses has been an easy jibe for opposition politicians since the NHS was founded. And perhaps there is some truth in these comments too. Things have moved a long way since the days when a hospital was managed by a medical consultant, a matron, and an administrator. This simple tripartite management model was of its time and would hardly be able to sustain the kind of activity that the NHS now has to support. Regional Health Authorities have come and gone. District Health Authorities have also followed the same fate. Now Strategic Health Authorities are under the spotlight. Given the political predilection for targeting the management and structure of the NHS, it would not be unreasonable to expect the current model to at least be subject to some serious tinkering and at worst be put through another complete reorganisation. What does not and will not change is the need to deliver clinical and social support services and a process to assess that requirement and commission appropriate services to undertake it.

But while the management of services has been constantly subjected to change, the actual delivery of healthcare, the patient–doctor interaction, in community or in hospital, has changed very little in the five decades of the NHS. The patient journey of Jimmy Rawthorpe would look pretty much the same whatever the administrative arrangements of the NHS that lay behind it.

The current major players in the NHS and their general roles and those in relation to the NPfIT initiative are described in Figure 3.1.

The role of Primary Care Trusts

General

Primary care is the care provided by people you normally see when you first have a health problem. It might be a visit to a doctor or dentist, to an optician for an eye test, or just a trip to a pharmacist to buy cough mixture. NHS walk-in centres and the telephone service NHS Direct are also part of primary care. These services are managed for you by your local Primary Care Trust (PCT).

PCTs are now at the centre of the NHS and they get 75% of the NHS budget. As

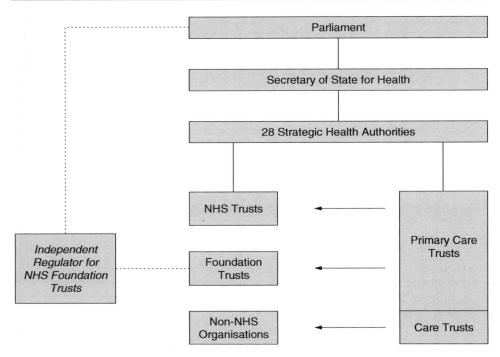

Figure 3.1 The NHS

they are local organisations, they are in the best position to understand the needs of their community, so they can make sure that the organisations providing health and social care services are working effectively. Your PCT will then work with various agencies including local authorities to ensure that the needs of your local community are being met.

For example, your PCT must make sure there are enough services for people within their area and that these services are accessible. They must also make sure that all other health services are provided, including hospitals, dentists, opticians, mental health services, NHS walk-in centres, NHS Direct, patient transport (including Accident & Emergency), population screening, pharmacies and opticians. They are also responsible for getting health and social care systems working together to the benefit of patients.

Before PCTs were established, there were Health Authorities who undertook this role and funding was routed through the Health Authorities to the GP practices and to the Hospital Trusts.

This latest organisational change has considerable implications for the providers of secondary services, as the PCTs can consider alternative models to support their local communities, i.e. they may decide to fund a community physiotherapist instead of always referring to the hospital physiotherapy department.

They could even fund community radiology image capture and contract with radiologists from another hospital or even another country to undertake the analysis. This phenomenon is known as 'shifting the balance of power', so that decisions made about the provision of local services are made locally.

This fundamental change in process was initially tried during the days of what was called 'the purchaser–provider split' with hospitals and GPs being providers and the Health Authorities adopting a purchaser or commissioner role. At this time, some GP practices were awarded GP Fundholding status, allowing them their own budget to invest, on behalf of their local clinical community, as they saw fit.

The new model gives this power to the PCT and ultimately their GPs.

NPfIT

The National Programme for IT does not provide *all* the funding for *all* the technology and support required to successfully deliver the objectives of the NPfIT programme. Considerable resources are required (both financial and people) to be provided locally. As the PCT is now the gatekeeper for 75% of the funding of the NHS, their role in enabling this 'local' provision of appropriate resources is key.

The PCT's role is also important in gaining maximum value from the NPfIT investment by ensuring the opportunities for a reconfiguration of services locally take advantage of the opportunities provided by the provision of advanced technology.

The role of Strategic Health Authorities

General

In 2002 the Government created 28 Strategic Health Authorities to manage the local NHS on behalf of the Secretary of State.

The health authorities have a strategic role. This means they are responsible for:

- developing plans for improving health services in their local area
- making sure local health services are of a high quality and are performing well
- increasing the capacity of local health services – so they can provide more services
- making sure national priorities – for example, programmes for improving cancer services – are integrated into local health service plans.

Strategic Health Authorities manage the NHS locally and are a key link between the Department of Health and the NHS. It is their responsibility to ensure central health policy, as determined by the Department of Health, is implemented locally. This function was previously undertaken by the 13 Regional Health Authorities, but these were considered to be too distant from the actual local delivery of healthcare services to be able to make appropriate decisions and efficiently monitor performance.

NPfIT

The five 'clusters' which are charged with ensuring that the national programme is successfully implemented are artificial organisations. They are *not* statutory bodies and as such have limited powers. It is the Strategic Health Authorities who will performance-manage the implementation of NPfIT and have a key role in prioritising the phases of development and implementation.

In addition, within their 'local' patch, they will act as facilitators, ensuring adequate resources are in place to enable a successful programme to be delivered.

The role of the Secondary Care Trusts

Acute Hospital Trusts

Hospitals are managed by Acute Trusts, which make sure that the hospitals provide high-quality healthcare, and that they spend their money efficiently. They also decide on a strategy for how the hospital will develop, so that services improve.

Acute Trusts employ most of the NHS workforce, including nurses, doctors, dentists, pharmacists, midwives and health visitors as well as people doing jobs related to medicine – physiotherapists, radiographers, podiatrists, speech and language therapists, laboratory scientists, counsellors, occupational therapists and psychologists. There are many other non-clinical staff including receptionists, porters, cleaners, specialists in information technology, managers, engineers, caterers and domestic and security staff.

Some Acute Trusts are regional or national centres for more specialised care. Others are attached to universities and help to train health professionals. Acute Trusts can also provide services in the community, for example through health centres, clinics or in people's homes.

NPfIT

Although NPfIT will provide the bulk of the resources for the implementation of core functionality and infrastructure, some of this will only be pump priming and each Trust will have to ensure there are adequate resources to continue funding this infrastructure after the first two years. In addition, it is anticipated that each Trust will provide resources during the first two years especially, with implications for the training of *all* employees in the adoption of these new clinical applications.

Foundation Trusts

General

Foundation Trusts are a new type of NHS hospital run by local managers, staff and members of the public which is tailored to the needs of the local population. Foundation Trusts have been given much more financial and operational freedom than other NHS Trusts and are reported to represent the Government's commitment to de-centralising the control of public services. However, these Trusts remain within the NHS and are still subject to the NHS's performance inspection system.

The first 20 NHS Foundation Trusts were authorised by the Independent Regulator and were established on 1 April and 1 July 2004.

On 26 July 2004, Health Secretary John Reid confirmed his support for 20 more hospitals to become NHS Foundation Trusts. He also confirmed that the next wave of NHS Foundation Trust applications is to be expanded to include, for the first time, three-star rated Mental Health Trusts. Currently only three-star rated Acute and Specialist Trusts are able to apply for foundation status.

How these Foundation Trusts, with their newly acquired autonomy, will fare with centrally mandated initiatives such as the NPfIT remains to be seen.

NPfIT

As with other Acute Hospital Trusts, Foundation Trusts will have to find considerable resources (people and money) during the early stages of implementation and a commitment to continue funding the ongoing costs of elements of the national programme.

Ambulance Trusts

General

There are 33 ambulance services covering England, which provide emergency access to healthcare. If you call for an emergency ambulance the calls are prioritised into three categories:

- Category A emergencies – which are immediately life-threatening
- Category B or
- C emergencies – which are not life-threatening.

The control room decide what kind of response is needed and whether an ambulance is required. For all three types of emergency, they may send a rapid response vehicle, crewed by a paramedic, equipped to provide treatment at the scene of an accident. Over the last five years the number of ambulance 999 calls has gone up by a third, with a large proportion of these being inappropriate calls.

The NHS is also responsible for providing transport to get patients to hospital for treatment. In many areas it is the Ambulance Trust which provides this service.

NPfIT

As with Acute, Mental Health and Foundation Trusts, it is anticipated that Ambulance Trusts will also have to contribute towards the cost of the implementation and ongoing costs of elements of the national programme – NPfIT.

Care Trusts

General

Care Trusts are organisations that work in both health and social care. They may carry out a range of services, including social care, mental health services or primary care services. Care Trusts are set up when the NHS and Local Authorities agree to work closely together, usually where it is felt that a closer relationship between health and social care is needed or would benefit local care services.

At the moment there are only a small number of Care Trusts, though more will be set up in the future.

NPfIT

At present, it is anticipated that all Trusts will have to contribute to the cost of any NPfIT implementation, although the central funding of the infrastructure by NPfIT will reduce the costs to the NHS considerably.

Mental Health Trusts

General

Mental Health Trusts provide health and social care services for people with mental health problems. Mental Health services can be provided through your GP, other primary care services, or through more specialist care. This might include counselling and other psychological therapies, community and family support, or general health screening. For example, people suffering bereavement, depression, stress or anxiety can get help from primary care or informal community support. If they need more involved support or treatment they can be referred for specialist care.

More specialist care is normally provided by Mental Health Trusts. Services range from psychological therapy through to very specialist medical and training services for people with severe mental health problems. About two in every thousand people need specialist care for conditions such as severe anxiety problems or psychotic illness.

NPfIT

As with other Trusts, Mental Health Trusts will be expected to contribute resources to the implementation of NPfIT (people and money).

Special Health Authorities

General

These are health authorities which provide a health service to the whole of England, not just to a local community – for example, the National Blood Authority.

Special Health Authorities have been set up to provide a national service to the NHS or the public, under Section 11 of the NHS Act 1977. They are independent, but can be subject to ministerial direction like other NHS bodies.

NPfIT

It is anticipated that Special Health Authorities will have to contribute to the implementation of NPfIT where it is applicable to their service.

The role of the Department of Health

General

The Department of Health supports the government to improve the health and well-being of the population. The Department is responsible for:

- setting overall direction and leading transformation of the NHS and social care
- setting national standards to improve quality of services
- securing resources and making investment decisions to ensure that the NHS and social care are able to deliver services
- working with key partners to ensure quality of services, such as:
  - Strategic Health Authorities, the local headquarters of the NHS
  - the Commission for Healthcare Audit and Improvement (CHAI) (now the Healthcare Commission) and the Commission for Social Care Inspection (CSCI), new independent bodies
  - the NHS Modernisation Agency and the Social Care Institute for Excellence to identify and spread best practice locally.

NPfIT

The Department of Health has negotiated with the Treasury for considerable additional top-sliced funds to support the implementation of NPfIT. Their role is to ensure NPfIT supports the NHS's modernisation agenda.

The ever-changing NHS

One of the major factors in delaying the implementation of any health-related IT initiative has been trying to build technology infrastructure on constantly shifting sands. We will see later when we look at an earlier IT programme – the Resource Management Initiative (RMI) – how a way of providing clinicians with clinical information to manage more effectively the use of resources and improve clinical outcomes, was hijacked into a scheme to provide information to monitor the new purchaser–provider relationship. This resulted in alienation of those clinicians who had put in considerable efforts to making the IT element of RMI work, only to see their efforts being misused in contract monitoring.

Monies intended for the implementation of *Information for Health* were likewise hijacked, with 70% of hypothecated funds being used to fund other purposes.

It might help to define some of the terms that the NHS uses when discussing the ways that systems are funded. 'Top-slicing', 'hypothecation' and 'ring-fencing' sound like terms from an inquisitor's guide book. Sadly their meanings are more prosaic. Most funding for the NHS is distributed from the Treasury through the Department of Health down to Health Authorities (and now Primary Care Trusts). Top-slicing means the money never filters through the local Health Authorities, but rather arrives at its destination direct. An example of top-slicing was in the early days of Medical Audit when considerable funds for Medical Audit were top-sliced and distributed directly to the Trusts.

Ring-fenced meant that there was money (that had not been top-sliced) but which nevertheless was intended to be used for some specific purpose(s) – in this case information management and technology (IM&T). In the first year of ring-fenced monies for IM&T, the waiting times pressures proved too powerful and broke down the fence. In the second year the rather grander sounding 'hypothecation' was intended to be a more robust ring-fence – but in practice was just as useless and these monies too were used for immediate shortfalls and not for the longer term IM&T investment.

The NHS is an organic structure and will always be changing its shape in order to deliver the appropriate support for a constantly changing population in an ever-changing world. It should not be perceived as failure for any long-term initiative to change its shape and priorities as the organisation it supports changes. What should not change, however, is the underlying desire to support the clinical process, in whatever form those processes evolve.

There has been some evidence that these fundamental objectives have been altered to what are perceived by many to be objectives with a political motive. That may well be the price we have to pay in order to get the commitment from the very top, and the secret is to accept these underlying motives and still derive the clinical benefit desired.

The National Programme is a series of important projects which are essential if the NHS is to change to support the delivery of healthcare fit for the twenty-first century.

To understand what the National Programme is trying to achieve and what it is having to work with, we must consider the historical developments, the foundations upon which NPfIT will be built.

So what are the foundations on which this monument is being built?

Chapter 4

Doesn't the NHS have computers already?

One of the founding fathers of the Internet, Paul Baran, (in an interview at the Charles Babbage Institute in 1990) has suggested that no one individual can claim to be the builder of a cathedral that takes hundreds of years to complete, as each generation adds a layer onto that previously built. It has been much the same with NHS IT. Sometimes the layers represent real systems out there in the hospitals or in the community, doing a real job of work; at other times the layers are initiatives or strategies, launched from time to time by the NHS, intended to kick-start the NHS into the computer age. The NHS Care Record Service (NHS-CRS) that is being built today was previously a strategy called the 'Integrated Care Record Service' (ICRS). This, as a strategy, is built on an earlier programme called the Electronic Patient Record (EPR) initiative, which in turn was built on the foundations of the Hospital Information Support Systems (HISS) projects and pilots. And before that there were countless Patient Administration Systems (PAS) and projects and pilots of every hue and complexity imaginable, from Resource Management to Nursing Care Planning systems.

'We are in a fashion industry,' a computer salesman told me once. 'Every year the NHS is out looking for the newest, sexiest, most eye-catching systems they can find, but they can never afford the whole outfit. So they accessorise here and there with a bauble or two, and next year the fashion will have moved on.' As an example of this 'gadfly' tendency, in the 1990s the NHS commissioned several pilot projects that were known as 'HISS' – where the aim was to see if every patient-based activity within a single hospital could be linked by computer. We will look at the achievement of HISS in a later chapter, but by most measurements HISS was a huge success. Hospitals in Greenwich, Darlington, Wirral, Burton, and Winchester proved that doctors and nurses would use a system that could deliver them with critical patient details at the bedside or in a clinic. Huge savings could be made in operational processes. Big benefits could be delivered in patient outcomes. The success of these projects should not have come as a surprise to the NHS, but it seems that they did. For by the time the systems were operational, the fashion had moved on. The NHS had lost interest in HISS and was starting to draw up plans for ambitious EPR pilots.

It is like chasing the rainbow: as soon as you approach it, it has moved on. You never get there. It has been a perennial problem. The NHS focus moves onto the next and newest fashionable initiative, and very often some good systems get left behind. There is barely a hospital where you will not find a passionate enthusiast who has written and developed a computer programme that will revolutionise the NHS. Or so he will tell you. He will demonstrate it to you and it will charm you with its ease of use, its captivating graphics, and its raw clinical potential. But then no one will deploy it. The developer's life is one huge frustration caused by the blinkered inability of the NHS to grasp the real potential of his extraordinary system. Even his own hospital has been lukewarm, funding just a limited pilot in one ward, and what is the point of that?

I've seen dozens of systems like this. The truth is, they are all good. Sometimes they really do work. Many have some limited commercial success. But strangely in a marketplace which includes over 400 acute hospitals, it is rare for even a commercially successful system to be able to claim more than a dozen user sites, and this creates new problems of its own. Unless the NHS is prepared to spend extravagant sums, then a customer base of a dozen sites does not give the developer a revenue base large enough to fund the growth and development that the system probably needs. So it begins to fall behind the glitzy systems coming in from the USA, and in time it is acquired by a predatory software vendor looking only for a user base into which it can sell its own application. And so the market fragments some more. But even big, experienced software vendors from America with thousands of user sites, and solid, proven systems, have never found the NHS an easy market to crack. The NHS is coy and battle-scarred when it comes to computer systems. They have become so used to blind alleys where huge budgets and whole teams have been devoted to systems that in the end, just didn't work, or were too slow, or were swept away in the latest Trust merger. Now they view every IT suggestion with distrust and suspicion that borders on the pathological. There are risk-takers in the NHS, but on the whole risk taking has rarely been a smart career move. So after decades of dabbling with IT, the NHS is starting to look less like a fashion model and more like a clothes horse, clad with a hundred loose and ill-fitting garments that don't match.

It was into this confused world that the National Programme for IT (or NPfIT as it is called) was launched at a conference in Harrogate in 2002. The delegates at the time were nonplussed. 'It will never happen,' was the regular response that I heard time and again from NHS professionals, used to the whims and fancies of government initiatives. But swiftly, like an army appearing out of the dark, it did happen. Huge budgets were approved, advertisements were placed, teams were mobilised, and the unstoppable juggernaut that was to become the world's biggest IT programme began to gather momentum.

So what actually is the NPfIT? What areas does it cover? What is unique about it? Is it worth the effort and resources? When can we expect to see what?

To understand NPfIT, we must appreciate and understand the history of what has gone before – from PAS to EPR and beyond. We need to position NPfIT in its correct place in the chequered historical landscape of the pilots and projects and national initiatives that preceded it.

Healthcare and information

The NHS is often described as the world's fourth largest employer, after the Chinese Red Army (reportedly over 5 million people), Indian Railways (1.6 million) and Wal-Mart (1.5 million). However you compare it, it is, as we have already discovered, a huge organisation, employing nearly a million people in the NHS in England and looking after the healthcare of 50 million people.[1] And let's face it, you don't manage an organisation like this without some serious IT. So the NHS has bought into computing, and it has been doing it for over 30 years, since the very early days of mainframe computers, punch cards, and paper tape. It has been, and still is, one of the biggest customers for computers in the world. There are at a reasonable guess over 20 000 major computer systems humming away in computer rooms serving the NHS today in hospitals, in GP clinics, in dental surgeries and offices. Who knows how many PCs the NHS has? In 2004 the NHS struck a new deal with Microsoft for operating system, desktop products and bespoke software for 900 000 PCs, compared to its previous allowance of 500 000.

Before NPfIT at the annual Healthcare Computing Show, held every March in Harrogate, over 200 companies would turn up to demonstrate their wares in a dazzling and bewildering shopfront of hardware and software and state-of-the-art devices. So there seems to be no shortage of solutions aimed squarely at the NHS. From the throng of suits in the hall and BMWs in the car park at the show, it would also seem that, despite being a frugal customer (in terms of the percentage of its income that it has devoted to computing), the NHS has nonetheless spent and spent well.

And so it should, because the NHS is in the information business. There is an easy way to prove this. Take the basement staircase in any major hospital and follow the signs to 'Medical Records'. If it is a typical hospital you'll encounter a locked door. But peer though the glass and you'll see around half a million manila folders packed onto maybe 15 miles or more of shelving. Information. Lots of it. Now head back upstairs to the X-ray department. Here you'll discover another huge store – this time full of enormous brown envelopes. It is the film store. Hundreds of thousands of X-ray films. Now head to A&E, or to Maternity. More records. More information. Drive down to your GP surgery and look past the smiling receptionist. Filing cabinets, full of records. The NHS, you see, is awash with information. It has been estimated that about one third of NHS time is spent collecting, distributing, storing, transporting or sharing this information. Or sometimes just looking for it. Medicine is a discipline that desperately, voraciously generates and consumes information. And that is why the NHS is such a big and effective user of computers.

Or is it?

Well, actually it clearly isn't that effective a user of computers or we wouldn't still have all those manila folders, and all those porters pushing trolleys full of files, and all those miles of shelving. The NHS may be one of the world's largest purchasers of IT systems and services, but IT has not always worked well for the NHS.

Consider the comparison we introduced earlier when we looked at booking your airline ticket:

Table 4.1

Booking a flight	*Booking a hospital appointment*
You or your travel agent searches online for the best day and the best route and the best price for you. Books it online.	Your GP writes a letter to a consultant at the local hospital asking for an appointment for you. The consultant replies, also by post, with a day that suits the hospital, but not you.
Time taken: 10 minutes	Time taken: Up to a month
Flexibility: Very high	Flexibility: None

Or think about this scenario. If you wanted to borrow money from your bank manager, you would expect her to look at a computer screen and have instant access to information about you before making a decision – whether to lend you the money or not. You might expect her to find answers there to some of the following questions:

- Who you are?
- What is your current state of finance?
- What are your financial commitments with the bank?
- What are your financial commitments to third parties?
- What is your income now and in the future?
- What are the risks?
- How can these risks be minimised?

Not a problem. The banks and building societies have been using technology to do this sort of thing since before Bill Gates was in long trousers.

But now imagine you are a patient in a hospital ward. A new doctor comes to your bedside to ask how you are feeling. You are not feeling well. Would you expect the doctor to be able to look quickly at a computer screen to see:

- Who you are?
- What is wrong with you?
- What drugs you are taking?
- What operations you have planned?
- What treatment regime you are on?
- What allergies and complications you have?
- What is planned?

Ahh. Well unless you are very lucky and you find yourself in one of the half a dozen or so hospitals that can do this, then it isn't going to happen. The systems aren't there. And neither is the data. So just hope that your medical notes are there, and that someone has got around to filing the letter from your GP and the handwritten notes from your consultant, because if they haven't, then your bewildered new doctor probably won't have a clue even what is wrong with you.

So let us begin by accepting that it would be a good thing for your doctor to have this information. More than this, it would also be a good idea to support these busy clinicians with tools to help them to diagnose and monitor your progress. That would improve your chances of a successful outcome. It would save the NHS money if you get better faster.

Most of us, used to watching ER on TV, would probably expect that this kind of technology is already in widespread use in the NHS. After all, computers have been with us for more than a generation.

How hard can it be?

Well there are several reasons that might help to explain why it has not happened yet, and it will help to understand them.

System purchases have been too fragmentary

This is certainly a reason. We estimated earlier that there are over 20 000 computer systems in the NHS. They come from hundreds of different suppliers and they all work in different ways. And no two hospitals have the same combination of systems. Typically there is very little integration between systems and even a single hospital may have up to 30 or 40 systems which do not share data at all.

Clinical information is complicated

This is true too. Clinical information can include images and sketches and handwritten scribbles, long text reports, difficult words, complicated distinctions, opinions, suspicions, shorthand comments, codes and numbers.

And for a long time there were no good standards for exchanging data in healthcare. And healthcare lacked a *common terminology* – so that you could never be sure if a medical condition with one name at your hospital would be called the same name at the hospital next door.

Computerising medicine is hard

Believe me, banking, retail and airlines are easy compared to medicine. Medicine does not deal in easy things like the balance of your savings account. It deals with complex data types, opinions and workflows. And if you get it wrong, then the impact can be very serious. Compare it with the kind of data exchange when you buy a plane ticket. There is actually very little data about *you* that is required to process your flights across the world.

A very different story if you are being treated for a medical condition.

Computerising anything is hard

History is littered with bad IT projects. Many millions of public and private pounds or dollars have gone down the pan. The Ministry of Defence spent £800 million on its Nimrod air defence early warning aircraft before realising the onboard computer system could not distinguish a Ferrari from a low-flying Russian fighter. More recently the same ministry budgeted £250 million for an ultra-secure head office computer system. Its final cost was £380 million and was described by some staff who refused to use it as 'the most expensive E-mail system in the world' (*New Statesman* June 27 1997).

There were problems, too, with the London Ambulance project,[2] and in the 1990s with an NHS project in Wessex.[3] It was an ambitious, far-reaching health IT project which attempted to get all users within the Wessex region of England (a swathe of geography stretching from Basingstoke to Dorchester, taking in cities like Salisbury, Portsmouth, Southampton and Bath) to use the same computer system. Years after the project was expected to be up and running, computers still lay in their boxes stacked up in offices. The project cost between £20 million and £63 million. According to the *New Statesman*, 'the exact figure is unknown because the authority failed to keep track of its money, some of which was spent on shower curtains and towels used by employees who jogged at lunchtimes'.

These experiences have lead to a nervousness among NHS Chief Executives when any suggestion about clinical IT rears its ugly head. No one wants their career blighted by a failed IT project.

The NHS is too big to computerise

Well it helps if you imagine the NHS as a whole network of separate businesses. There are around 300 hospital trusts – and each of these is about the size of a FT-100 company, with around 2000 employees, and a turnover measured in the £100 millions. There are thousands of GP practices – and each of these is like a small business. And all of these organisations have been busily doing their own thing with IT for years. Imagine trying to implement a system into several hundred companies simultaneously, each of whom has a system already that they are perfectly happy with, thank you, and you will understand why no one has tried it before.

The NHS is resistant to change

While this attitude is not peculiar to the health sector, tried and trusted ways of working provide a comfort blanket in a sector where change can bring increased risk. Resistance to change may prove to be one of the biggest obstacles to the success of NPfIT, as we shall explore later.

There has been a lack of investment

In 2000, the Prime Minister (who at that time was under pressure over NHS performance) promised to increase overall spending on healthcare to the EU average by 2005.[4] Figures at that time suggested that the European average spend on healthcare was 8% of gross domestic product (GDP) – GDP being a rough measure of the wealth of a country. The UK's health spend was calculated as 6.8% – which was well below the average. It meant we were being beaten on this important indicator by every European country apart from the Republic of Ireland.

In real terms, this promise meant that the government would eventually have to find an extra £2.56 billion or so every year. If inflation in the NHS runs at 2% a year, the total budget in 2005/6 would have to be at least £77.5 billion – compared with £48.5 billion when Tony Blair made his promise.

Coupled to this information was the fact that NHS spending on IT was considerably less, as a percentage of total expenditure, than any other major industry. A report in 2002 by Derek Wanless[5] identified funding problems as a key reason for the lack of and poor use of IT in the health service, and recommended a doubling of investment in IT.

A Government White Paper, *Information for Health*, published in 1998 made a strong case for increasing the amount spent on NHS IT. It argued that 'the NHS cannot afford *not* to make the investments necessary to deliver this strategy'. Despite this, however, the NHS consistently failed to make available specific additional funds for the implementation of IT. Attempts to top-slice specific IT funding failed; attempts to ring-fence specific monies for IT failed; attempts to provide 'hypothecated' funds failed. The failure was caused by these funds being raided for non-IT purposes in an environment of intense pressures to reduce overspending. It seemed that *Information for Health* had failed too. It had failed to convince the NHS Chief Executives who had yet to see the potential for IT.

Doctors are too busy to use it

Doctors and nurses are already ridiculously busy. We know that. So imagine asking them to use a computer to record clinical information, request X-rays and order lab tests. Unless the system is so slick that it actually makes life easier for them, they probably won't bother. To date, many of the clinical systems that have been introduced are complex, difficult to navigate around and are not clinician-friendly.

This in turn results in the doctor shouting to the nurse, 'log onto the computer and just order me some blood tests will you?' while they rush off to their next patient.

This has a twofold effect: first, it adds additional workload onto the already busy nurse; and second, it reduces the potential clinical benefit of using IT – to provide decision support and information to the doctor during the requesting process.

The NHS has been too busy piloting new systems

This has been a particularly curious phenomenon. It would be hard to imagine any organisation investing continually in new pilot projects without ever planning to take any of them forward. Yet it is hard to resist the conclusion that this is exactly what has happened with the NHS. For the last 20 years we have seen sporadic injections of project money into countless pilots, with very patchy results. 'Pilotitis' has become an endemic condition, with nearly all hospitals and Trusts at some time undertaking a pilot for some clinical IT project or other, but with very few making it beyond the pilot stage.

Pilots, of course, are fine if they really are intended to be research & development – that is, when they really are trying to answer an unanswered question about a wholly new IT approach. But very few seem to fall within that definition. Most seem to be set up to answer just one question – can we start this project on the cheap and then persuade our Trust to spend more on it later?

But the trouble with this question is that the answer is nearly always 'no'. So why bother? If there is already evidence of benefit for the implementation of clinical IT, in whatever form, then what is a pilot telling these hospitals and Trusts?

Take for example electronic prescribing. There is a raft of evidence to support the benefits of supporting the prescribing process with computers (we'll look at some of this later). You no longer need a pilot to tell you this. You can go to the literature. Bringing clinical decision support into the complex prescribing process reaps huge clinical and financial benefits. The evidence is out there, mostly from the US but also from the UK, that this investment is worthwhile. So why have over 30 NHS Trusts undertaken pilots of electronic prescribing? Was it to prove benefits that were already proven? And what happened to these 30 pilots once the pilot period ended? Well, unfortunately, regardless of whether the pilot was successful or not, they very rarely ever turned into full implementations. Why? Well the answer turns out usually to be pretty simple. It is because the Trust didn't have the money for a full roll-out of the technology. So why, we might ask, do the pilot in the first place?

When a lot of effort and resources are invested in a pilot which does not result in a complete implementation, those involved become increasingly frustrated and cynical. Those not involved will see the lack of a roll-out being due to the pilot being a failure. So before embarking on any clinical IT project, it should be assumed that it is for a complete implementation, that the funding is available for a complete installation and the 'pilot' is actually Phase 1 of a trust-wide implementation.

In conclusion, the reasons why the NHS has been less than successful in its attempts to computerise are many-fold. That isn't to say it is not possible, but all these factors must be considered when attempting to modernise.

Chapter 5

The legacy

Once, of course, it was all done on paper. Armies of typists worked for the NHS typing out laboratory reports and ward summaries and clinic lists and discharge letters and all sorts of documents that are now effortlessly printed out by computers.

Or else it was done with handwriting, and even today if you take down a volume of notes from the shelf in any medical records library, you might be astonished by the number of handwritten notes and slips and forms, scribbled diagrams and margin comments that still populate those manila folders. Ironically, it would probably have been easier to introduce NPfIT into an NHS with no computers at all than into one which already has over 20 000.

The best of the HISS pilots, as we will discover later, were often the ones (like Greenwich Hospital) that took a site from 'Day One', with virtually no computers at all, directly to a day when all activity was computerised. Sites with a patchwork of existing systems bring extra problems – problems of migration of existing data, of retraining, and of the loss of well loved functionality. These are the systems that the National Programme for IT calls 'the legacy'. They may be very old systems, cranking away on monochrome terminals, long overdue for replacement. Or they may be last year's most exciting fashion system – a dazzling multimedia power-tool of computing luxury and brilliance. Or probably, they will sit somewhere inbetween, quietly doing the job they were bought to do. They are all part of the legacy.

The word 'legacy' was never intended to be a pejorative term. It does not imply that a system is old-fashioned, or non-compliant, or no good at what it does, even though it is often used that way by the acolytes of NPfIT. A legacy system may be long overdue for replacement. Or it may be fresh out of the box. Some legacy systems (for example Laboratory Management Systems) are not included within NPfIT. Others (like Patient Administration Systems (PAS)) are. Either way, it is still an issue for NPfIT. All legacy systems will need some measure of compliance with data-sharing standards if the whole programme is to work – even those that are not directly included in the programme.

And many legacy systems will have to be swept away and replaced, however good they may be. The question of the legacy hangs over everything, and the ability of the big service providers to handle the transition of the legacy may be the biggest challenge they face.

The legacy in the NHS is wide-ranging and very complex. It has grown by surviving wave upon wave of national and local initiatives, and by developing ways to meet the ever-changing demands of an evolving NHS. We shall see later how IT programmes, initiatives and fashions like PAS and HISS and RM and EPR and PACS and ERDIP have swept through the NHS since the 1970s. All have left their mark.

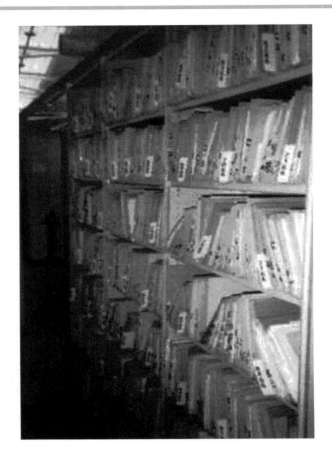

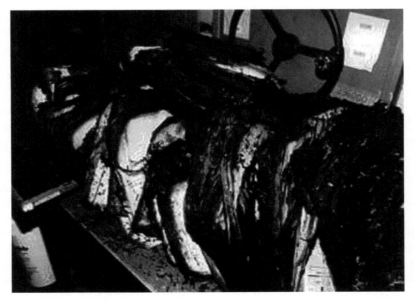

Figure 5.1 Medical records

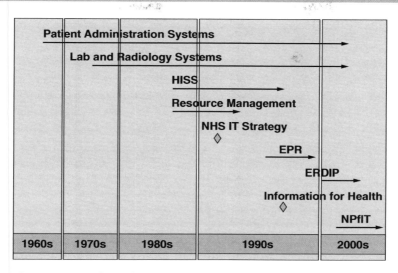

Figure 5.2 Timeline of NHS IT projects to date

Like an evolutionary tree, however, not all have survived.

Huge projects like the 'Resource Management Initiative' of the early 1990s have been and gone and barely a ripple remains. Most of the computer systems, for example, purchased under that ambitious programme (and there were hundreds) have long ago been quietly switched off. Today's legacy systems in the NHS are the evolutionary survivors of this headlong process. It has been a case of survival of the fittest, and the systems that are out there today, the legacy, are there because they have proved themselves. They have survived. In computing terms, the NHS Trusts and GP practices who own them have found it worthwhile to continue to pay for their operation and maintenance, and this in turn suggests that they must be doing useful jobs.

This section looks at the legacy. What are the systems that are already out there, and what do these systems do?

Patient Administration System (PAS)

Hospitals have been using computers now for 30 years, but mostly in the non-clinical areas such as finance systems or administration. The most used system is the Patient Administration System (PAS) which allows clerks to schedule appointments and generally 'manage' your various trips to the hospital outpatient clinics and your occasional inpatient stays.

Doctors and nurses can sometime be a bit dismissive about PAS systems. 'I've never found anything useful on our PAS system,' they will tell you. They are probably right. But they may be expecting a little too much of the PAS. PAS was never designed to be a clinical computer system. It was never designed to hold information about your medical condition, or notes from your GP. What it was designed to do is manage the business of a hospital, and this is something that it does exceptionally well. The humble PAS system, that started life as a dull clerical recording system hidden in the basements of hospitals, has emerged to become the unlikely success story of NHS computing. Today no hospital in Britain operates without a PAS. It would be unthinkable. The PAS tracks and manages

Master Patient Index/Demographics					
Clinic Appointments	Clinic Modules	Waiting List	Clinical Coding	Live Bed State	Casenote Tracking

Figure 5.3 Patient Administration System (PAS)

all the patient-based activity of the hospital. It manages the busy schedule of outpatient clinics that nearly every hospital operates, it tracks patient notes, monitors waiting lists, and keeps note of which patients are in which ward. This may seem like mundane stuff, but it is the very lifeblood of a hospital.

Although the PAS is not normally designed to hold any *clinical* data about patients, there is usually one important respect where this rule is broken. At the end of your clinical episode, a coding clerk will assign a clinical code to your episode, describing what you've had done and what your final diagnosis was. We will look at coding in more detail later on in this book, but at this stage the fact that a code has been recorded which identifies what was wrong with you, and what procedures you had, is a powerful source of data for managing the whole of the NHS. It is the PAS that collects the Hospital Episode Statistics (HES) that enable the DoH to monitor activity between hospitals, and in future, it is expected that each individual named consultant's clinical data will be accessible on the Internet. When this happens it is essential that the quality of clinical coding is of the highest order.

GP systems

You've probably noticed that your GP practice has a computer. Most do. GPs have been among the most pioneering users of IT. But it hasn't always been that way. For a while it looked as if there was no place in the high street surgery for computing of any sort. GPs were too busy, they couldn't afford the technology, and the benefits were dubious.

Then, in 1982, the Minister for Information and Information Technology announced a scheme to promote the use of IT in general medical practice.

As a carrot, the Government would pay for 50% of the cost of purchasing and installing a microcomputer system in 150 practices. It was a great incentive that would kick-start computers into GP practices. Another initiative came from two of the GP system suppliers. They gave away free systems to GPs in return for the use of the clinical data collected. This data they would then sell on to drug companies – with the patient identifiers removed. It was a clever business model, and it worked, for a while. GPs began to embrace computers.

Other incentives included the *Working for Patients*[1] reforms, which required practices to record and analyse events occurring to their patients and measuring outcomes. And an even better incentive came in the 1990 contract for GPs, linking their earnings to their success in meeting government targets for activities like child immunisation, screening of the elderly and carrying out cervical smear tests. This was a very good reason to install systems which enabled GPs to record these events and produce invoices for payments.

The Oxford Community Health Project (OXMIS) pioneered the use of computers in general practice during the early 1970s, with registration and contact records for more than 100 GPs being held on a mainframe computer, enabling the generation of activity and management data for the GPs together with epidemiological data. Records were coded using the OXMIS Codes – the first comprehensive primary care coding system, predating the Read Codes now used by most NHS practices by more than 10 years.

So GPs have been using clinical systems for decades and in many cases they are far more computer-literate than are their acute hospital colleagues. Several (or even many) GPs have been prescribing electronically for years.

One thing you shouldn't lose sight of: GPs are small independent businesses, so convincing GPs of the value of NPfIT means: What's in it for them? Why should they bother? What are the benefits – to them or to their patients? What does NPfIT give them that they don't already have?

Over time the choice of GP systems settled down to one of four main suppliers – AAH Meditel, In Practice Systems (IPS), Torex and EMIS – but dozens of other systems survived, and today there are probably more than 20 systems in regular use.

Pathology laboratory systems

Whenever your GP or your specialist asks you for a sample – usually of blood or urine, but sometimes of sputum, or perhaps a cervical smear, or a wound swab or any other sample of tissue or fluid – then the pathology laboratories are where the sample will end up for examination. The role of the pathology laboratories in the NHS has evolved from fairly humble beginnings in cramped one-bench labs to the modern, well equipped and technology-rich environments we see today. The labour-intensive work practices of 20 or 30 years ago inhibited growth in this diagnostic arena, but in recent years, the introduction of high-speed complex analysers has resulted in the service's rapid growth, and with it an increasing dependency by the clinicians on the service it delivers.

It is poignant to remember how rapid the change in this service has been. As recently as the early 1970s pregnancy tests were performed by injecting a mouse with a patient's concentrated urine for five consecutive days. Afterwards the mouse was gassed, and the tissue was extracted and weighed! There was little requirement for computers in that process. The skills that those laboratory technicians required then are a far cry from the competencies expected of the biomedical scientists who are now the personnel in the pathology service.

In the UK, the laboratories deliver a diagnostic service. The doctor gives clinical information to the laboratory and requests a series of investigations. The laboratory undertakes those tests (and in addition any others they think the clinical information or results suggest). There has been an increasing dependence on pathology investigations for diagnosis and monitoring of clinical episodes.

In this process, the way that the NHS works can be markedly different from the way that, say, hospitals in the USA will work. One American approach to diagnosis may be to ask for a battery of common investigations before the specialist even sees the patient, prior to taking any clinical history. The results are then used along with the clinical history to help the doctor make a diagnosis. This model can be seen in one-stop shops or walk-in centres. However, when the patient does see the doctor (later that same day) there is an increased likelihood of coming away from that single session with a diagnosis and course of treatment agreed.

The move towards lab-testing nearer the patient (e.g. at the GP's practice, in a walk-in centre or even at a chemists) will require a new delivery model for the laboratory services, a model more aligned with the American laboratory service. This new model will require modern laboratory systems and although these systems are 'additional services' in the NPfIT portfolio, they are an essential component of the evolving NHS.

In the pathology labs of the twenty-first century, the increasing use of robotics will reduce the time-consuming tasks. They will reduce the need for centrifugation of samples (a current bottleneck in laboratory workflow), with specimens being separated (serum/plasma from cells), sorted and dispatched to appropriate testing laboratories without human intervention. This is science fact and is already happening in many high tech laboratories. The samples may even be sent to other countries for analysis and results passed electronically back to the requestor. This potentially changes the entire workflow model in diagnostic services.

It is a fair assumption that the diagnostic service will continue to be core to the delivery of healthcare, regardless of the way in which the service is delivered. What will not change is the laboratories' total dependence on reliable computer systems to support their work, linking complex analysers to the laboratory workflow systems.

> There are external forces bearing down on the traditional hospital-based providers of laboratory services. There is a drive to provide more community-based services which are more convenient for the patient. This includes diagnostic services in DTCs, home testing, increased over-the-counter products and the potential for testing facilities in retail settings, such as pharmacy outlets. Will these services be part of a planned integrated pathology service, or separate to it? These are issues that cannot be ignored by pathology today.
>
> Dr Ian Barnes, National Director of Pathology Modernisation

Radiology and PACS systems

Nearly every hospital has a Radiology Information System, although relatively very few (yet) have a PACS. The Radiology Information System (RIS) supports the management of a patient requiring an X-ray or other image. The system allows the Radiology Department to schedule an appointment, providing a key to link that appointment and subsequent image to the patient's ID and history. The workflow within the department is supported by the RIS, culminating with the report of the investigations being assigned to an individual patient and forming part of the radiology record for that patient.

And just as digital cameras have been replacing old-fashioned film for our holiday snaps, so in Radiology there is now the opportunity to dispense with traditional imaging methods that use expensive film and chemicals and move to a new era of digital images. The system which allows this transition is known as PACS – Picture Archiving and Communication System. As part of the National Programme for IT, all Trusts will have a PACS by 2008.

PACS and RIS together bring huge benefits to both radiology departments and the wider clinical service. These previously prohibitively expensive systems are now affordable, thanks to the bargaining power of the national programme.

What brings real benefits is the ability to distance the interpretation of an image from the site where that image was captured. It means that the specialist doctor who is able to interpret that faint shadow on your X-ray image no longer needs to be in the same room as the film. In the future, images could be captured in the community without the patient having to go to hospital, and that image transmitted for interpretation anywhere in the world.

Simply implementing PACS into the current healthcare model will not result in maximum benefit. But using PACS and the infrastructure provided by NPfIT to redesign the provision of radiology services will bring untold benefits to clinicians, radiologists and patients alike.

Theatre systems

To understand what a theatre system does, we must first understand the work-flow in the operating theatres.

There are three elements to a patient's journey in an operating theatre:

- preparation
- operation
- recovery.

In the preparation phase, the patient is given the necessary drugs and prep work prior to being wheeled into the theatre.

In the theatre itself, the patient is monitored by the anaesthetist whilst the surgeons and theatre staff undertake the operative procedures.

The duration of any operation is not always predictable and although a guesstimate of operating time can be made in a large percentage of cases, some will overrun and others will underrun. As you might imagine, this makes definitive scheduling of theatre time almost impossible.

Then once the patient's operation is completed, they are wheeled into a recovery bay where they are constantly monitored prior to being sent back to the ward for post-op care.

In each of these three stages, the theatre system provides support through scheduling resources, actively monitoring progress and recording outcomes and interventions. The theatre system can then be used to produce an operating theatre report which is sent with the patient to the ward and included in their paper notes.

Data collected during these three phases of the patients episode is also available for clinical audit and for legal purposes.

Nursing and care planning systems

Computer-aided nurse care planning systems were introduced as part of the Resource Management Initiative in 1986. Up until this time, nurses charted the planned care, targets and anticipated nursing interventions on a ward-based paper Kardex system. The plan was paper-based, handwritten and only available in one place at one time, usually in the ward or in the sister's office.

At the time when resource usage in hospitals was being identified in order to support clinical management, the use of computers in the nurse care planning process was considered. It was agreed that as part of the RMI, every hospital would procure a nurse care planning system with a nurse staff-rostering system. In time these two elements would become a single system which was anticipated to enable better planning and scheduling of the nursing resource to the care plan.

Throughout the RM Initiative, all hospitals would and did procure and implement computerised care planning systems. The systems required that nurses identified targets and interventions from a database library and assembled them into an individualised computerised care plan for each patient. The selling point to the patients was that they would receive a care plan specifically tailored for them and that the printout of the care plan would be available for all who came into contact with them (including relatives and the patient themselves), making them aware of what was planned and when. The paper care plan would be updated by the nurse as and when interventions had been successfully achieved.

Considerable effort had to be put into setting up the databases of interventions, goals and objectives, in order for the system to work. Because of the lack of appropriate infrastructure, however, it was rarely possible for the nurses to view the electronic care plan at the patient's bedside. This meant that the plan had to be printed onto paper. And because the plan was on paper, any changes were made on the paper plan and not directly onto the computer. This resulted in the paper plan becoming part of the legal record of care and as such was subject to the rules of retention – i.e. the paper care plans now had to be stored (like all medical records) for a minimum of seven years. Hospital ward cupboards were stuffed full of care plans long after the patients had been discharged.

The process also resulted in busy nurses having to queue for access to the one ward-based computer system to update the care plan (usually retrospectively).

It was a classic example of what can go wrong even when intentions are good. In principle, what was attempted was laudable. However, because of the technology available at that time, the concept of computerised care plans was always doomed, and the systems became no better than simple word processors.

In time almost all care planning nursing systems were switched off and became another element of what we will later see as the 'failed' IT component of the Resource Management Initiative.

There is a new reincarnation of the idea, however, within the National Programme for IT, as we shall see later. Integrated Care Pathways are the latest descendant of these early care plans, widening their scope to include all clinical practitioners and not just nurses. However, these too will fail unless they can be accessed and updated at the bedside. NPfIT intends to implement the infrastructure to support this.

Accident & Emergency systems

The NHS, as we have discovered, is in the information business. All around a hospital you might find information stores with shelves full of patient records.

One of those places might often be in A&E. For practical reasons many A&E departments prefer to keep their own records about your encounters, rather than adding the paperwork to your main medical notes down in the medical records library. Often there is a good reason for this. The medical records library may be a long way away. It might take a long time to find and retrieve your notes, and A&E necessarily has to move fast. So many A&E departments have become mini-hospitals in their own right, managing their own record stores, and these days running their own computer systems.

A good A&E system won't try to duplicate all the data that is held on PAS (although many do). It should have a link to PAS so that when you arrive clutching your bleeding knee they can quickly find out who you are and book you in. Then the system will manage your 'triage' – which is where a nurse will quickly assess how urgent and life-threatening your condition is. It might run a calculation algorithm against observations that the nurse will make and will assign a triage category that may decide, for example, that your torn knee is less urgent than the condition of the patient who came in after you. Then the computer has to monitor your waiting time – this is for national statistics – but it also helps the department to spot if anyone's wait is unreasonably long. And finally it allows details of your treatment to be recorded. You may have seen, in many A&E departments, a large whiteboard where nurses scribble up patient names and cubicle locations. This is an important part of any A&E department because it enables the doctors and nurses to see where each patient is as they move from waiting room to X-ray to examination room. Modern A&E systems usually have a computerised version of this whiteboard. Some even go so far as to give each patient a badge with a radio transponder that tracks the location of every patient all the time. That kind of technology is still rare in the NHS, but the benefits it can bring are substantial. Just think of the stories about patients who have passed out in the toilet and not been discovered until too late.

Most hospitals now have an A&E system, or else use an A&E feature on their PAS. Integrating A&E will be one of the early objectives of NPfIT.

Maternity systems

Maternity systems manage the collection of a whole set of very special data associated with pregnancy, birth and early infancy. As a specialty, of course, maternity is a rather unique area. Unlike other specialties in a hospital, the women who pass through maternity departments are not normally ill, so strictly speaking we shouldn't even think of them as patients. In fact they are usually particularly healthy young people. But pregnancy exposes mothers to risks and complications. And of course this is one specialty where the hospital will hope to admit one person but to discharge two. It is all a little complicated.

Maternity systems need to manage and monitor the progress of mothers and babies through the hospital. They need, for example, to bring in serial measurements from ultrasound examinations to allow midwives and specialists to calculate the risks of conditions like Down's syndrome. They have to cope with multiple attendances and home care. They must keep records of previous pregnancies because complications with a previous baby might affect a later one. Critically, they have to allow a whole range of complicated assessments to be entered: general health checks, gynaecological examinations and a wide range of antenatal, birth, and postnatal examinations of mother and baby.

Most maternity hospitals and maternity wards in general hospitals have some level of computing capability already. Many have a dedicated maternity system. Others might make do with some limited additional functionality on the PAS.

Other specialist systems

The NHS-CRS will provide the technology to support most clinical functionality. This might include ordering laboratory investigations, requesting radiology images, prescribing drugs, ordering food and transport. It will also provide a mechanism for capturing clinical information which will form the patient's record of care.

However, as currently envisaged, the basic NHS-CRS might not have, in the early stages, the specialty-specific components for, say, ophthalmology or cardiac care, or oncology, or audiology, or any of the other -ologies that make up the medical specialties of a busy hospital. These historically have been provided by specialist, and often separate, systems. They are not usually large systems. Very often they may have only a single terminal. Neither are they especially complex in their operation. They collect data and they store it, display it and report it. What makes them special is the very particular knowledge that they contain. They've been written and designed, almost always, by doctors – specialists in their particular field. They collect information on eyes or ears or knees or liver parasites in exactly the way that this consultant or that consultant wants the information collected. They are, in a real sense, repositories of clinical knowledge. If you were to take an audit of all the computer systems in any large hospital today, you might be surprised by the number of these little clinical computers that lurk in departments all around the hospital – often sharing information with no other system, not even the PAS. One London hospital, at a recent count, had over 40 such systems. One of the objectives of NPfIT is to see an end to these. It isn't that they don't do a useful job. It is more that they don't share the information they collect with anyone beyond the small team of people who use them. One of the challenges for NHS-CRS will be to find a way that will allow the knowledge and genius wrapped up in these systems to find a new home in NPfIT. It may not be easy. Failure to do so will have the potential to leave the NHS with too many islands of information, and this brings increased clinical risk and wastes valuable resources.

Chapter 6

Learning from history: what NHS IT projects have told us to date

If history repeats itself, and the unexpected always happens, how incapable must Man be of learning from experience.

George Bernard Shaw (1856–1950)

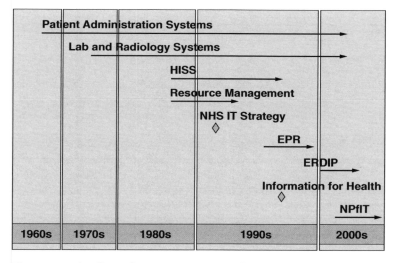

Figure 6.1 Timeline of NHS IT projects to date

As we have already concluded, computerising the delivery of healthcare services is a complex process. That IT brings benefit is not disputed and there have been countless examples of successful IT projects in the NHS. However, moving relatively small successful projects into mainstream delivery has not been achieved to date.

We have just heard about the existing 'legacy' systems: mostly departmental and stand-alone clinical specialty systems. There now follows a description of a number of initiatives aimed at integrating these separate systems together, and the conclusions we can draw from them.

Local efforts can build upon the cumulative experience of several generations of partial successes, and learn to avoid some of the more severe difficulties.

McClenahan (2000)

What we have had is a large number of fragmented projects with varying degrees of success. This section focuses on the genesis of the NPfIT NHS Care Record Service (NHS-CRS) in the last 20 years.

The HISS projects

Perhaps the boldest of all NHS initiatives before NPfIT was the so-called 'HISS' project. HISS is an acronym for 'Hospital Information Support System'. It was, perhaps, a poorly thought out acronym, lending itself to inevitable headlines that cried, 'Boo HISS'. The name at least, however, was not the invention of the NHS. HISS came from the USA, and in the late 1980s doctors began arriving back in Britain after spending time practising in hospitals across the Atlantic, and they started to draw unfavourable comparisons between the systems that they had used in America – and the ones that they were expected to use (or more often were *not* expected to use) over here. Small working groups were sent on fact-finding missions to the USA to see how things worked. And so the HISS initiative was born, and launched in 1988 by the NHS Executive. It was a cautious launch. Three procurements would act as pilots for the technology. A new team – 'the HISS central team' – was formed, and massive multi-volume requirements were sent out to interested vendors. The UK IT industry had never seen anything like it before – at least not in healthcare. In a sense this was probably intentional. After all this wasn't a procurement directed at the UK IT industry. This was a search for an unashamedly American solution.

When the first contract award at Greenwich General Hospital was announced in 1990, there was a sharp intake of breath from the media. The contract was awarded – as expected – to the Atlanta-based software company HBO & Company – soon to become part of the giant McKesson corporation of San Francisco. But it wasn't the fact that the contract had gone to the Americans that caused the shock. It was the value of the contract – a reported £8 million. Today we might consider this all fairly small change when compared to NPfIT – and in fact the costs of NPfIT (depending upon how you count them) would more than pay for three HISS systems of this size for every hospital in England. But this was an innocent time when computers were seen as a luxury in medicine, not as an essential tool of the profession. Since 1988 the NHS has spent £56 million on the HISS initiative. This includes £48 million in financial support to 16 projects at 25 hospitals. Of this, some £32 million was spent on the three main pilot projects, at Nottingham, Darlington and Greenwich.

The initiative was intended to support the NHS reforms by exploring ways in which integrated computer systems could provide the information needed by NHS acute hospitals. Integrated hospital computer systems cover all aspects of a hospital's functions and management, and are linked together so that information is entered only once and shared by authorised staff across the whole hospital. Such systems typically include links between the systems we met in the last chapter, the Patient Administration Systems, departmental systems such as Pathology and Maternity and administrative systems to facilitate clinical audit and research. They may also include electronic ordering of clinical tests and the transmission of the results of those tests.

The National Audit Office (NAO) undertook a review of the HISS initiative,

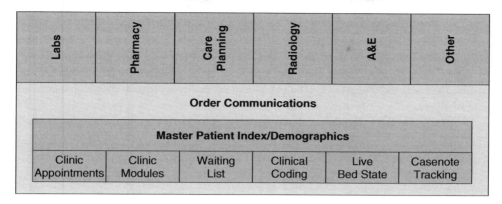

Figure 6.2 Hospital Information Support System (HISS)

reporting finally in 1996,[1] examining the progress of six projects funded under the initiative. This is a summary of what they found:

Hospitals with one project:

- Darlington Memorial Hospital NHS Trust
- Greenwich Healthcare NHS Trust
- Nottingham City Hospital NHS Trust
- Kidderminster Healthcare NHS Trust.

Hospitals participating in a consortium in East Anglia:

- Addenbrookes NHS Trust
- James Paget Hospital NHS Trust, Great Yarmouth.

Hospital participating in a consortium in the West Midlands:

- Birmingham Heartlands Hospital NHS Trust.

The NAO report made the following main points on the progress of the project:

> When the initiative was launched, there was limited experience of integrated systems in the NHS, and the NHS Executive wished to explore the costs and issues involved in implementing such systems.
>
> The NHS Executive selected the three main pilot projects within two months, to make early progress in support of the NHS reforms. Judged by today's standards, most of the hospitals visited by the National Audit Office were not ideally geared up to undertake a complex computer project when their projects were selected. A number of the deficiencies were addressed during procurement or implementation.
>
> There have been significant delays in implementing key systems and in completing each of the six projects examined by the National Audit Office . . .
> - Two of the projects had been reduced in scope, deferring the completion of the projects and delaying the achievement of cost savings and quality improvements.
> - Five of the six hospitals had kept within budget. However, slippage had delayed the achievement of cash savings for all of the projects.

- By March 1995, the projects had achieved cash savings of £3.3 million (8% of lifetime savings) compared with the £10.4 million (25% of lifetime savings) originally expected by that date.*

*Projects had been justified on the basis that quality improvements would outweigh the net cash cost. The hospitals examined considered that their systems had brought about improvements in the quality of service.

The Report concludes that the NHS Executive might have achieved greater value from the Initiative had they been able to proceed at a slower pace at the outset. Although the projects have experienced problems along the way and had not delivered benefits as quickly as originally hoped, the Initiative had provided lessons from which the NHS could learn, and these early systems should not be seen as indicative of what might be expected by hospitals embarking on integrated systems today. But there is still much work to do to ensure that integrated computer systems play a full part in the development of the NHS reforms.

Looking at this conclusion today, it reads like a Civil Service fudge. 'There wasn't enough time. The scope was wrong. The savings weren't what we expected. We should have done it slower. There are lots of lessons to learn.' But did they learn any of the lessons? One lesson they might have learned was that although the projects took longer than expected, they did work well in the end. Another lesson may have been that there were too many software solutions chasing too few pilots. A bit of rationalisation might have helped everyone. Soon after the HISS pilots were implemented, and well before the NAO's 1996 report,[1] the NHS had begun a stampede towards HISS systems, driven not by the NAO report, which was notoriously late in arriving, but by the anecdotal success of HISS in the early pilots and by the arrival of high-pressure salesmen from far and wide with HISS solutions to sell. It could have been a goldrush time for the right solution – but it seemed as if the right solution just didn't quite exist. Lots of companies entered the fray, but success was always measured in ones and twos, frustratingly too few to support the infrastructure of analysts, developers and implementers that a product as bewilderingly complex as HISS undoubtedly required.

HBO & Company, for example, should have been in pole position following the success of their American built 'Star' system at Greenwich. But they found the NHS an uphill struggle and it took several years to consolidate their position in the HISS market with more takers for 'Star' at Trusts like Solihull, Walsall and South Ayrshire. Oracle Corp with their development from scratch at Nottingham seemed to run out of steam. McDonnell Douglas with their Australian 'Homer' system at Darlington brought their development over to Warrington in Cheshire, and had some early successes with a string of wins in East Anglia and Scotland. But by the end of the 1990s they too were running out of enthusiasm for this stubborn marketplace. Another American system, TPA (The Precision Alternative) from First Data, found a home at Kidderminster and another at the Central Middlesex Hospital, but went little further. A system from Utah-based GTE was installed at Birmingham Heartlands, but nowhere else seemed to want it. At the same time Wirral, Bath and Winchester were busy implementing the American

TDS system, while Burton and Sunderland were racing ahead with yet another US software system from the Meditech corporation of Massachusetts, and Dudley Hospital was busy deploying a solution from New Zealand developers IBA. It seemed as if everyone who wanted to experiment with HISS had to try something new.

Before many years had passed, yet more vendors and more software packages would join the fray. Vermont-based IDX corporation would start an ambitious clinically led project at Chelsea and Westminster – a project that would later play a major part in helping them to win two-fifths of the NPfIT NHS-CRS software contract; Kansas-based Cerner, a US market leader, would lobby hard to enter the NHS market and would embark on projects in North London at Chase Farm and North Wales at Conway and Denbighshire. They would go on to be the core software providers behind 'Choose and Book'. McKesson, the giant US successor to HBO & Company, would introduce a new Australian HISS system, MedTrak, finding takers at the Royal Infirmary of Edinburgh, Bury & Rochdale, and in Norwich; Canadian arrivals PerSé would begin a big HISS project at Preston, and Capula Elan would find takers for their Saudi Arabian-developed 'Oasis' HISS at sites like Dunfermline and Brighton.

By this time any acute Trust that didn't have a HISS was trying to find a way to afford one. While the authors of the 1996 NAO report were valiantly fudging their conclusions, much of the NHS was procuring systems regardless. The HISS systems that started to flood into the NHS in the wake of the HISS pilots weren't all American or Australian. Maidstone-based developers System C found a strong following for their 'Medway' system and began a string of contract wins that began to shake the resolve of the Americans, taking in Aintree Hospital in Liverpool, Swindon, Tameside and Christie Hospital in Manchester, among others. An early in-house development at Hammersmith Hospital would go on to become a successful HISS for Dublin-based IMS, with further implementations at Trusts like Blackpool and St Helens. UK-based SMS (later Torex) would become the biggest HISS supplier in the country by building on the strength of their PAS user base. Their proposition was a HISS that could be incrementally added to the existing PAS. It was an idea that worked well and won dozens of converts from Perth and Kinross down to the hospitals in South West Thames, taking in major sites like the Royal Liverpool Hospital, Manchester Royal Infirmary and Sheffield's Northern General Hospital.

With hindsight, of course, it should have been obvious that this plethora of solutions was not the best way to computerise the NHS. Too many vendors were left vainly trying to support tiny communities of users – often numbered in twos or threes. The procurement process, instead of discouraging this absurd diversification, seemed well designed to fuel it. Overseas software vendors soon learned that they had to 'buy' their way into the NHS. This meant that the first contract win would have to be made at a knock-down price – possibly even at an operating loss to the company. For software developers this sort of grand gesture is quite easy to make. After all, your software only really costs the price of the DVD that it is recorded onto. You can give software away here and there in the hope that you will win contracts later. But it is a perilous game. Software is not, ultimately, a free good. Eventually someone has to pay. The trouble was that the software companies all had over-optimistic views about the success that would follow their first cheap sale, and what happened in practice was that someone was always ready to undercut them when the next opportunity came around. The inevitable outcome for the NHS in the mid-1990s was that almost every project was underresourced, and almost every software suite was underdeveloped.

As the NAO discovered, implementing integrated HISS systems is not easy. Healthcare is a stubbornly difficult process to computerise. Despite the surge of interest in HISS, by October 1995 less than one quarter of the 260 acute NHS Hospital Trusts in England had HISS systems implemented or under development. This number had not increased significantly by the start of the NPfIT programme.

It is important to understand HISS if we are to make head or tail of NPfIT. In many ways, NPfIT is a direct descendant of the HISS project. Many of the concepts pioneered by HISS are firmly part of NHS-CRS: order communications, integrated applications, a single patient record – all these were tested and proved by HISS. The extraordinary thing about the HISS pilots was really that it took so long before anyone sat back and recognised how successful they had been. Greenwich Hospital was live in 1991, demonstrating to regular parties of NHS visitors just how effective a single, hospital-wide information system could really be. Today the old Greenwich Hospital has closed, but the system lives on at the new Queen Elizabeth Hospital in Woolwich. It remains perhaps the best computerised hospital in the NHS, a claim that might only be challenged by Burton Hospital in the Midlands or Wirral Hospital in the North West. Today at the Queen Elizabeth Hospital any doctor can access virtually all the clinical data on their patients, including laboratory results and X-ray images, at the click of a mouse. And it was achieved at a sum that will be dwarfed by the costs per hospital of NPfIT.

In our trawl through the history of NHS initiatives, by the way, Wirral and Burton (both referred to above) do deserve more than just a passing mention. These were early HISS users that became users not as a part of the centrally sponsored HISS initiative, but in spite of it. Neither were part of the centrally funded projects; both managed to find a way to fund the technology off their own backs; and both were startlingly successful. Their success was almost an embarrassment to the HISS team since the systems they chose were not from the same software suppliers as the HISS pilots. Wirral bought a system from Atlanta-based TDS Corporation (now Eclipsys) and Burton went for a system from Massachusetts-based Meditech Corp. The software may not have been the same but the principles were. The systems all did more or less the same thing, albeit with different screens and databases. The critical message that was eventually learned from these two sites – and from the HISS pilots – was that HISS worked.

Resource management

Not every IT initiative of the 1990s was as successful as HISS. One programme that the NHS might prefer to forget was also starting just about the same time as the centrally funded HISS initiative was getting underway. In 1986 a Department of Health 'Health and Social Security Notice' HN(86)34 announced an extension of the 'Management Budgets Programme' that was to be renamed the 'Resource Management Initiative'. It was the beginning of a bold, expensive, but ultimately ill-conceived plan that was destined to galvanise the energies of NHS IT departments for years to come. Six pilot sites were named. These were to continue the work of Management Budgets Programme's objectives to 'give better service to its patients by helping clinicians and other managers to make better informed judgements about how the resources they control can be used to maximum effect'.

The six Resource Management Initiative pilot sites were:

- Freeman Hospital, Newcastle
- Clatterbridge Hospital, Wirral
- Arrowe Park Hospital, Wirral
- Royal Hampshire County Hospital, Winchester
- The Royal Infirmary, Huddersfield
- Guy's Hospital, Lewisham and North Southwark.

The purpose of this bold new programme was to re-engineer NHS management processes by getting clinicians involved in the management structures of their hospitals. But this meant that there was a need to establish new management structures, and underpinning that restructuring came a requirement to collect structured clinical and financial information.

There is a story told about the birth of the Resource Management Initiative which may or may not be apocryphal. According to the story, by the late 1980s Prime Minister Margaret Thatcher was determined to slim down the costs of healthcare in London by closing down one or more of the city's hospitals. This much seems to be a matter of record. Everyone agreed, at the time, that London was overprovided with hospitals. So the Iron Lady asked the inevitable question: which one should we close? There was silence around the cabinet table. To the ideological economists of the cabinet the answer should have been obvious – close down the most inefficient hospital. But there was a problem. Which one *was* the most inefficient? Someone in the Department of Health drew up a table of costs that looked like a promising basis to choose the sacrificial site. It was immediately clear from the table that some hospitals spent vastly more than others. Even when you took account of the number of beds, a hospital like the Royal Free Hospital in Hampstead appeared to cost significantly more than its near neighbour The Whittington Hospital at Archway. Closing down the Royal Free, a showcase modern hospital with an international reputation for clinical excellence, was not, however, a politically palatable option. What Mrs Thatcher wanted to do was to close down the old workhouse hospitals because surely these were the least efficient, and politically the furore would be more muted. The health economists seemed to offer a glimmer of support. The reason that hospitals like the Royal Free cost so much more, per patient, to operate was not because they were less efficient. It was because they had a more difficult case mix. Take note of that term – 'case mix'. At the beginning of the 1990s that simple two-word explanation (soon concatenated to a single word – 'casemix') was put under the spotlight.

Intuitively it seemed like a reasonable explanation. Of course a modern teaching hospital would take more difficult cases than a humble district general hospital. And naturally these cases would be more expensive to treat. But did this difference in case mix really account for the huge disparities in hospital spending? What was needed was a way to measure case mix so that ministers could confidently compare the hospitals in London and select the most inefficient for the axe.

But again there was a problem. At that time, there was no process in place to accurately (or even inaccurately) measure the cost of each episode of care. There were very few IT systems in use in the NHS, and those IT systems that had been implemented were considered computers for 'The Management', and were therefore viewed with a degree of scepticism by the clinicians. (This scepticism, incidentally, has not entirely disappeared.) It meant that no one could go to the Prime Minister with any supporting evidence that would identify even a single hospital that cost more, for a similar case mix, than another. Impasse.

The real problem, of course, was bigger than the problem of choosing a hospital in London that could sensibly be shut down. It was a problem of management. How could the NHS soundly manage its huge budget if no one could really explain what it was all spent on? The Resource Management Initiative was the government's solution to this problem. It was not primarily invented as a computer project. It began as an exercise in change management and organisational restructuring. Nonetheless the implementation of a 'casemix' computer system was at the heart of this change, and the budget to fund a casemix computer at every hospital soon became the most visible part of the initiative.

The 'casemix box', as it became colloquially known, was conceived as a central database at each hospital fed by data from a host of feeder systems. These feeder systems would include the central Patient Administration System (PAS) and departmental systems like the pathology laboratory systems, of which there were often more than one in a single hospital: theatres, nursing care plan and staff rostering systems, A&E, radiology and pharmacy stock control. These feeder systems would submit an extract of defined data every night into the case mix database.

In principle, as each event, test or procedure was costed, this accumulation of data around an individual patient could enable an accurate resource usage to be calculated – and this in turn would enable the total costs of running the hospital to be attributable to the sum of individual patients or the resources used

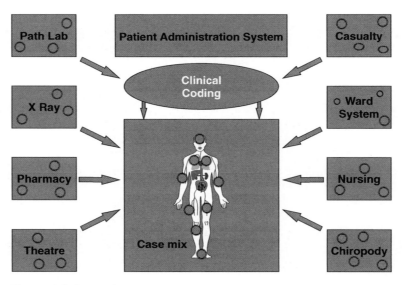

Figure 6.3 Case mix

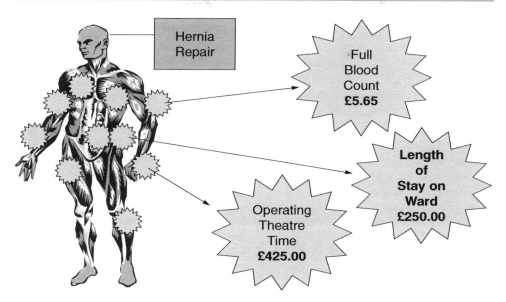

Figure 6.4 Resource management costs

aggregated into groups of patients (i.e. all diabetics; all inguinal hernia repairs, etc.). It was the Holy Grail of healthcare management, a data source that could explain why exactly the Royal Free Hospital cost so much more to run than the Whittington.

The vision of the 'casemix box' was that anything that happened to a patient in a hospital would be costed, and could be attributed to an individual patient and to individual carers. If you came in for a hip replacement operation, then all the materials and staff time and overhead costs that went into providing you with

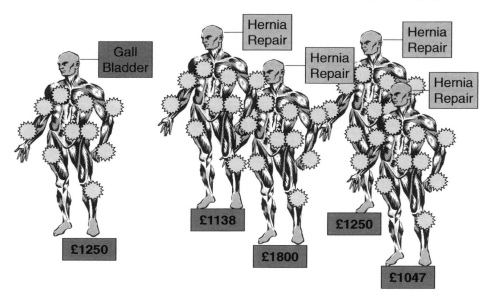

Figure 6.5 Assigning costs to a diagnosis

your new hip would be accurately tracked, so that at the end of your episode of care an accountant would be able to tell the NHS exactly how much your operation cost. If you had extra X-rays, or expensive lab tests, or stayed more than your expected number of days in a hospital bed, then all this would be there in black and white. It would be like billing but without the bill. Knowledge would be power. The hospital, armed with all this new information, would better manage resources, and changes in workload activity could eventually be compensated for by additional appropriate resources. That was the plan.

With all this data, the casemix system would allow all sorts of information to be distilled which was never available before. How much did a hip operation cost in Plymouth compared to the same operation in Grimsby? Did people living in cities suffer from more cancers than people who lived in the countryside? Was one method of treating angina cheaper than another? The opportunities seemed to be limitless. All this data could be assembled around a single patient, or patients grouped by operation, diagnosis, place of residence and more. The health economists were understandably excited.

The Resource Management Initiative was not itself a failure. Hospitals were successfully restructured as planned. The programme led to the directorate model that is now commonplace in the NHS, with clinicians playing a key role in the management of hospitals as clinical directors and directorate members. But the IT component of the initiative was, ultimately, a failure. Almost every Trust tried to do it. They took the money that was on offer from central funds, and they struggled to implement the systems. For a while there were hundreds of systems – hundreds of projects, thousands of interfaces, and thousands of data entry clerks painstakingly entering data into the shiny new computers. But still the initiative failed. Despite the millions of pounds spent on the IT, almost every casemix box was eventually switched off and left to gather dust. Why?

Why did Resource Management fail?

The evaluation of the Resource Management Initiative, undertaken by the Health Services Management Unit of the University of Manchester on behalf of the NHS Management Executive in March 1996,[2] concluded that the objective of engaging clinicians in management was a success. However, it concluded, the IT component, or casemix, failed.

Strange as it may seem, the Resource Management Initiative was not a part of any National NHS IT strategy. It was led by the finance directorate at the Department of Health. The IT component required a considerable resource commitment from the centre (Department of Health and Social Security), with each hospital having at least a £1 million allocation for the initiative, including a casemix database, and yet was not linked to any national IT strategy.

In total, over the three years of the programme, nearly £300 million was invested in the Resource Management Initiative – more than £1 million per hospital involved in the programme. There were a number of reasons identified in the evaluation that could explain why the IT element failed. Integrating the feeder systems to the casemix was problematic and very few sites managed complete integration. This meant that, in order to feed the casemix box with the data that it needed, hospitals began to employ low-paid data entry staff whose job it was to painstakingly type the data in – often, ironically, copying data from a computer printout generated by one computer into another that resisted successful integration. The technology was expensive and bulky. Casemix was retrospective and was considered a data collection exercise with little real benefit to the clinicians that were expected to 'feed the beast'. This was a feature of the Resource Management systems that is often overlooked. They were not, in any sense, operational. They didn't do a job of their own within the hospital. They were parasitic systems, feeding on the data collected by any number of real operational systems, or typed in by reluctant operators. The data collection was retrospective. It was not real-time, up-to-the-minute data. And this meant that the data analysis was also retrospective and not real-time. It made the casemix box a data store that would only ever be useful in generating data extracts for managers. It could never be reliably used by clinicians to help in the care of their patients, unless they were comfortable looking at data that would always be at least a day old, and a day in healthcare, like a week in politics, can be a long time.

A key component of the programme, for example, was the necessary introduction into hospitals of new nurse care planning systems. These nursing systems were intended to provide additional data to the casemix about nursing interventions, essential if managers were to get an accurate understanding of resource usage. But the implementation of these systems did not deliver any real-time clinical benefit for the busy nurses who had to use them. Nurses considered them a data collection exercise which they could ill afford to do. Any employee who has ever had the chore of completing endless paperwork that they will never see again will probably empathise with the nurses. Updating the database became a low priority, and the casemix system began to suffer from a shortage of data. What became apparent then, should, in hindsight, have been blindingly obvious from the start. Casemix was of no value to managers unless all the data was there, but this was an almost unattainable goal, if the system was not used in real time in the delivery of clinical care. It needed effective interfaces from effective systems and committed users prepared to feed the data in. When the casemix systems died they didn't die of old age. They died of neglect.

All this was unfortunate because a major new change was being introduced to the NHS in the 1980s and 1990s that would badly need the casemix data. This was the introduction of 'contracting'. The establishment of a purchaser–provider relationship between Health Authorities and GP Fundholders (these were the Purchasers) and hospitals (the Providers) resulted in a radical redirection of the use of casemix data. Now it was needed to provide the data required for agreeing and monitoring newly introduced clinical contracts. It was another demand for the casemix data, but it further removed it from the initial objective to 'give better service to its patients by helping clinicians and other managers to make better informed judgements about how the resources they control can be used to maximum effect'.

Although some may argue that the purchaser–provider relationship was itself an attempt to force healthcare providers to be more accountable for services delivered through the contracting process, the change in emphasis was not appreciated by the clinicians, who saw the use of their clinical data in this way as being, once again, 'for the management'.

If the demands of contracting weren't enough to breathe life into the ailing casemix computers, there was yet another NHS programme in the 1990s that should have done so. This was Medical Audit. It was the start of a project that would eventually measure clinical outcomes, that would measure the performance of one hospital against another, of one procedure against another, of one surgeon against another; it was a data collection programme that would lead inevitably to the new millennium of hospital league tables and star ratings. It was clear that Medical Audit and casemix were sibling programmes, despite the fact they originated from different government committees, and there were two ways that hospitals could go. Some sites forged a link between Medical Audit and casemix, and others didn't. Those that did, had more success. By using the casemix to provide clinical information in support of this new Medical Audit initiative which attempted to get clinicians to evaluate critically their clinical processes, there was more buy-in by the clinicians themselves. However, when the refocussing occurred due to contracting, even these sites began to lose that advantage. In the end all that was left was the sound of casemix boxes being switched off.

It is interesting to note that one of the initial six pilot sites, Arrowe Park Hospital in Wirral, delayed the start of their involvement in Resource Management until they had successfully installed their HISS. Their reasoning was that casemix should use data captured as part of the clinical process and should not be a separate exercise. This attitude led to some criticism from those attempting to centrally manage the RMI, but it turned out to be the correct decision. Casemix (and in the same way the electronic patient record) could not be delivered successfully until real-time integrated clinical support systems were being used. Without HISS, casemix was putting the cart before the horse.

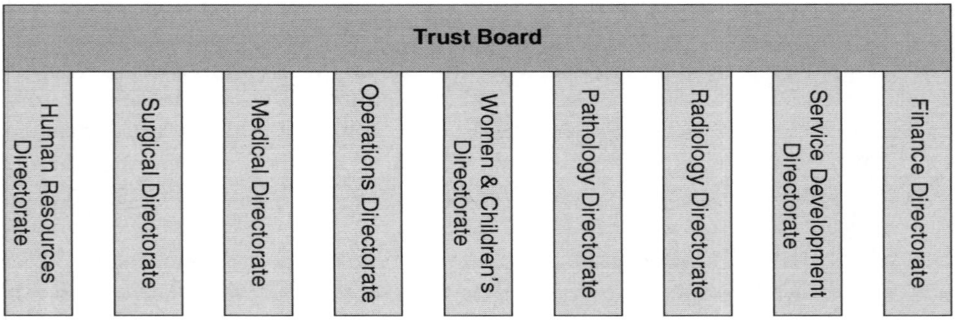

Figure 6.6 The new directorate model

So what was left for this fated scheme? Well, it wasn't all negative. On a positive note, the successes of RM were all around. There had been successful change management and restructuring. The initiative had seen the evolution of hospital directorates. In addition, a massive culture change happened in the hospitals. Clinicians began working more closely with non-clinical staff, and began to engage with IT. And this set the scene for programmes which followed. Crucially too, by some measures, the government quietly abandoned plans to close down a major London hospital. Supporters of St Bartholomew's Hospital, an East London Hospital that could trace its history back to 1123, and that had been openly threatened with the axe, could breathe freely – for a while at least. The new Labour government of Tony Blair swept into power in 1997 and there was no more talk of hospital closures. Intriguingly, there have been dozens of hospital mergers, and it hasn't been unknown for two hospitals to merge and then to move to a single new site. But that is another story.

As this book goes into production, there is a fundamental redesign underway of the way in which data is submitted to 'the centre' for performance monitoring of care delivery. A project called 'Revision of Waiting & Booking Information' (ROWBI) was established in 2000. The recommendations of this project[3] included a radical rethink of the way in which data is collected, that it should be patient-centric and of use locally, not simply collected for central monitoring purposes. All information should be about a single patient – when they saw the GP; when the GP referred; when the hospital accepted the referral; when the outpatient appointment is; when an inpatient admission was booked – and should be collected locally. In addition to collecting information about demand, the ROWBI report recommends that a parallel process identifying the available capacity should be undertaken. Demand would then measured against capacity. Queries would be run by the local hospital or PCT or even the Department of Health against this standardised data. It would not be a series of forms submitted by the local Trust asking 'How many patients are currently waiting for treatment?'

Why mention this here? Because in order to calculate capacity and demand of the services, you need to have information about lengths of stay, by procedure (i.e. operation) or diagnosis. If you have 36 patients on your waiting list for a hip replacement operation, and you know how much theatre time is required for each of these patients, and have a projected expected length of stay, you can then begin to intelligently schedule the care they require. And guess what? This is exactly the kind of data that the Resource Management Initiative's casemix was trying to collect.

The IT component of Resource Management Initiative was ahead of its time. As Wirral showed, the basic IT infrastructure of a HISS must first be in place and supporting the real-time delivery of clinical care *before* any attempts are made to capture clinical information into a data warehouse, or for that matter, an electronic patient record.

There is one postscript to the RM programme which has still to be recorded. While the stampede for HISS led to the arrival in Britain of a dozen or more solution vendors and a bewildering proliferation of systems, casemix, curiously, did not have the same impact. There were very few 'off the shelf' products that the Americans could bring to bear for this peculiarly British application. Instead, the challenge was taken up by more focussed UK developers, and by none more successfully than a small team at consultants KPMG. In 1994 KPMG started a healthcare IT business to sell its software to the NHS, riding on the wave of funds provided by the RMI. They succeeded famously. Four years later, in 1998 with casemix beginning to fail, the managers of this health business negotiated a management buyout from KPMG. It should have been the bursting of a bubble, but the small new company had big ambitions. They set off with a new vision and a great new name. With no real track record of operational NHS systems, with no experience of HISS, with no departmental systems in their kitbag, with no international presence, they set out to take on the Goliaths like SMS (later Torex) and HBOC (later McKesson) who had plenty of staff, international backing, proven products, and solid user-bases. Who would have bet that within five short years this minnow would have seen off almost every predator on its patch to become the core NHS-CRS solution provider for three-fifths of the NHS in England? The great new name that the new owners devised for their company in 1998 was iSOFT.

The 1992 NHS IT strategy

In 1992, the NHS published its long awaited IM&T Strategy.[4] It was a far-seeing document, and it laid down a number of key principles and initiatives, most of which have found their way into NPfIT. The key principles were:

- **Information should be person-based:** Person-based systems should hold a healthcare record for each individual which can be referenced to that person's NHS number. This may seem like an obvious principle today, but many systems in the 1980 had been based more around the organisation than the patient. Many pharmacy systems, to this day, are more concerned with recording what has come and gone from the storeroom than what has been administered or prescribed to a patient.
- **Systems should be integrated:** Wherever practical, the IM&T Strategy argued, data should be entered on a computer only once. Subsequently it may be available, in whole or in part, on other designated NHS systems. Steps should be taken to protect confidential information from unauthorised access. This was a principle that was to become fundamental, but it would take over a decade to become commonplace.
- **Information should be derived from operational systems:** This was a key principle, and also one that took the NHS a while to grasp. Subject to safeguards to maintain the confidentiality of personal health information, data should be obtained from systems used by healthcare professionals in their day-to-day work. There should be little need for different systems to capture information specifically for management purposes.
- **Information should be secure and confidential:** Great care should be taken to ensure that the information held on computer will be available only to those who need to know it and who are authorised to know it. This principle is rarely challenged, although it represents one of the toughest challenges for NPfIT.
- **Information should be shared across the NHS:** Back in 1992 this must have seemed like a visionary principle. Common standards and NHS-wide networking were proposed to allow computers to communicate so that information could be shared (subject to appropriate security of course).

The initiatives of the 1992 IM&T Strategy were:

Facilitating progress through projects

The Strategy should be supported by national facilitating projects. The Hospital Information Support Systems (HISS) project was seen as the major hospital project.

Developing an IM&T infrastructure

NHS-wide information sharing was to be facilitated by a national infrastructure, created through a number of components which reflected national policy. Local IM&T strategies would need to incorporate these components:

- **A new-format NHS number:** If you live in England you should, in theory, have a NHS number. This is the unique number that identifies you. To link a patient to information held about the patient on different databases by different organisations within the NHS requires a unique identifier common to all the databases. But there was a problem. The old NHS number had many formats which could not reliably be validated, and this has meant that many NHS organisations just didn't use it. This old number is gradually being replaced by a new 10-digit unique person identifier number where the last number acts as a check digit to guard against typographical error. Since July 1995 every newborn baby has been allocated a new NHS number, and everyone's old NHS number has been replaced with the new number.
- **Shared NHS Administrative Registers:** The NHS Management Executive agreed that shared population registers should be regarded as part of the national information systems infrastructure. There would therefore be a national approach to building such registers, based on agreement of all parties and led from the centre. These national NHS population registers would contain only administrative details about individuals such as name, address and NHS number. Clinical details would not be held. Hence they have been called 'NHS Administrative Registers' (or NHSARs).

  The register holds administrative data only and not information about clinical care or the health of individuals. Nevertheless, the confidentiality of the information that is held on the NHSAR must and will be maintained.
  - **people:** name; title; alias; sex; NHS number; alternative ID; date of birth; date of death
  - **links:** guardian role; address type e.g. home, student, etc.; address; registration (GMS); obstetric services; contraceptive services
  - **places:** address; postcode; geographic area
  - **organisations:** organisation type e.g. FHSA, acute provider; practitioner name/role in organisation.
- **A system of NHS-wide networking:** In 1993 an NHS-wide networking strategy was approved that resulted in major changes within the NHS. Problems of security of information on networks had led to much of the media attention paid to this network, known as NHSnet, but there are wider implications of these changes. NHS-wide networking does not refer solely to a computer network transferring text and numbers. The focus was on communication between organisations within the NHS using any form of media and method of communication including voice, image and mobile communication. Access to the NHSnet was strictly controlled and only organisations who had succeeded in applying for the NHSnet Code of Connection were allowed access to NHSnet.

  Additional financial benefits would be achieved by providing this networking infrastructure centrally (nationally) because of purchasing power of the NHS.

- **A thesaurus of coded clinical terms and groupings:** One of the key initiatives of the 1992 IM&T Strategy was the proposal of an infrastructure that would include a thesaurus of coded clinical terms and groupings to enable clinical information on signs, symptoms, diagnoses, preferred terms, synonyms, abbreviations and prescribed medication to be translated and understood on computers across the NHS. These clinical terms would include those used by public health doctors. The thesaurus was planned to have significant impact for people who were entering information onto computers or aggregating and analysing data from several sources. Clinical coding was also seen as a help in tracking health treatments and health outcomes and understanding patterns of morbidity.
- **A set of national standards for computer-to-computer communication:** Transferring encrypted data in a structured format from one computer system to another requires electronic data interchange (EDI). The method of EDI chosen by the NHS was known by the acronym EDIFACT (Electronic Data Interchange for Administration, Commerce and Transport), which at that time was a global standard for EDI administered by the United Nations and approved by the International Organisation for Standardisation.

  Without standardisation of these messages, the receiving computer would not know where to store the data items. EDIFACT sends a structured message in a predetermined and nationally agreed format which can then be automatically imported into a receiving computer from the transmitting computer.
- **A framework for security and confidentiality:** Sharing of information across the NHS raises issues of security and confidentiality. A national framework was proposed in the IM&T Strategy to ensure that users would have access only to information they were authorised to know and needed to know.

  All staff would be expected to respect security controls, such as passwords, and to ensure that personal health data is properly safeguarded. Breaches of confidentiality would be subject to disciplinary action. Great care would also be taken to ensure physical robustness and security of hardware and software.

Maximising value for money

The 1992 IM&T Strategy provided a framework that aimed to ensure that the NHS would get the best possible value for money from expenditure on computer systems.

Enabling people

The Strategy also included plans for training and developing people to apply IM&T imaginatively and effectively.

NAO report on the 1992 Strategy

Sir John Bourne reported to Parliament[5] on the National Audit Office's review of the £152 million IM&T Strategy, not including expenditure in the wider NHS. The report also covered the new IM&T Strategy (*Information for Health*) launched in September 1998.

Sir John reported that the NHS Executive's '1992 Strategy' successfully communicated a vision and a set of basic principles directed at the overall aim of providing information about patients to enable the NHS to deliver better healthcare. NHS organisations visited in the course of the study said that the Strategy had given direction to local IT developments. They also welcomed some projects designed to translate the vision of the Strategy in to practice.

However, Sir John concluded that:

- a lack of overall objectives contributed to a lack of direction in implementation;
- while the Executive set objectives for individual projects, their business cases were not always complete in terms of specific, measurable and time-related objectives, financial analysis and proposals for monitoring and evaluation;
- the Executive did not consider how all the projects related to each other, and overall, the Strategy lacked coherence;
- the impact of the strategy was limited because NHS bodies were not always clear about the purpose of projects and because of problems with their sequencing; and
- the Executive had not yet fully evaluated the impact of all the key projects.

1992 IM&T Strategy Projects

The Integrated Clinical Workstation project (ICWS)

One grand NHS IT initiative of the old millennium was the Integrated Clinical Workstation (ICWS) project. The clinical workstation project was initiated in the early 1990s as a means of ensuring clinicians could access easily computer technology in order to work more effectively.

The NHS Centre for Coding and Classification (NHSCCC) was established in 1990 and it was they who instigated the Integrated Clinical Workstation Project. Its aim was to produce a detailed clinical user requirement and several prototype demonstrators to illustrate this, and show how information required by practitioners might be collated and used in an integrated way. It was envisaged that this would maximise the opportunity for the Clinical Terms Project by providing and allowing practitioners to capture data in a useful and meaningful manner that would not interfere with the natural flow of their work

The project had some degree of overlap with what was later proposed through the EPR programme and did not focus specifically on the design aspects of the user interface, but was established with a broader remit on the adoption of computer technology in support of clinical care.

With hindsight it might have been more advantageous if the Clinical Workstation project had addressed issues such as a common NHS-wide user interface, and common icons. In its early stages, this project was intended to concentrate on ensuring that nurses and clinicians could interact with computers easily, using their own clinical terms. Additional projects were also initiated to develop information systems for GP practices, DHAs, FHSAs and communities. One example might be the Community Information Systems Project (CISP) that was set to run in parallel with HISS. It was intended to ensure that, for example, hospital information on the discharge of patients would be passed directly to community systems, subject to security and confidentiality safeguards.

In 1999, the ICWS project was managed as a parallel project alongside the Electronic Patient Record Programme, but there were several areas of overlap between the two programmes which resulted in confusion in the NHS as to which project was delivering what.

As discussed later the projects should have clearly defined objectives and focus, to minimise project creep and duplication of effort and resources.

The EPR programme

So we come to the programme that perhaps, more than any other, set the groundwork for the National Programme that was to follow – in tone if not in scope. The Electronic Patient Record programme was set up to shift the balance from the use of computers to help managers with administration, to the use of computers to help clinicians give better care to patients. The programme was focussed on the acute sector and it was anticipated that the outcome would influence the development of the next generation of IT systems which would be in general use in five to seven years from the start of the Programme.

The Electronic Patient Record Programme 1994–97 identified an incremental model for the development of an Electronic Patient Record. This built increasing functions onto the basic IT support of departmental systems and PAS, reinforcing the philosophy of supporting clinical care with IT. By using IT to support clinical care, a 'passive' record of that care would be automatically produced.

It was a natural evolution of the HISS programme, and a distinction was made between these integrated real-time clinical support systems (known as the 'active' elements of EPR) and the output from these systems (known as the 'passive EPR' or 'the record'). Data for secondary analysis (previously attempted as part of the RMI) would also be captured in a data warehouse as a by-product of the active systems.

So the EPR had three components:

- integrated active clinical support systems
- a 'passive' record
- data warehouse for secondary analysis.

You have to see the EPR programme in the context of what had gone before. To date the NHS had had 10 years of varying sluggish success with clinical and non-clinical IT, culminating in a number of HISS sites and a failed casemix initiative. The EPR programme tried to build on that. It identified a pragmatic model which enabled all hospitals to identify where they currently stood with their clinical IT and how to move from their current position to one which would support a paperless electronic record. To this end, a six-level model was agreed which was proposed by the EPR Demonstrator Sites and the Manchester Health Services Management Unit of the University of Manchester, who were undertaking an evaluation of the EPR programme. The EPR levels of functionality, now part of the folklore of NHS computing, would be added to these base systems as follows:

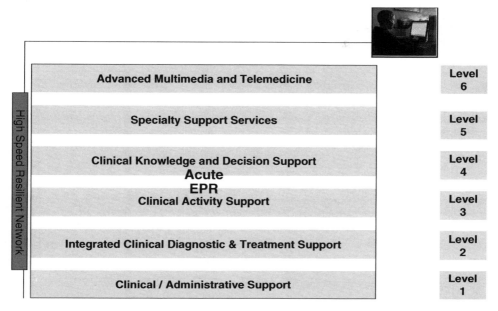

Figure 6.7 The EPR six-level model

EPR level 0–1

The main characteristics of this level were:

- partial implementation of PAS
- limited casemix/EIS analysis
- departmental systems limited to Pathology, Radiology and Pharmacy but not integrated to PAS.

For this level, a full PAS consisted of MPI, inpatient management, outpatient (OP) clinic management, waiting lists, case note tracking.

EPR level 2

The key characteristics defined for level 2 were:

- full implementation of PAS, including availability at ward level and in departments
- data warehouse (casemix)/EIS systems
- full range of departmental systems integrated to the PAS.

EPR level 3

This approximates to level 2 but has additionally:

- virtually full order communications/results reporting
- extensive integrated departmental systems
- some clinical systems

- care planning and multidisciplinary care
- (early) electronic prescribing.

EPR level 4

For level 4 the key characteristics were:

- complex electronic prescribing
- development of clinical decision support
- workflow and imaging begin to appear
- integration of specialist clinical systems common
- paper case notes still used as prime source.

At the time that the EPR programme was published, no sites in the NHS could claim to be delivering functionality that would meet level 4. It was an ambitious target.

EPR level 5

For level 5 the key characteristics were:

- full electronic patient record available
- clinical decision support/rules
- extensive workflow
- case notes no longer stored in paper form – electronically available in real tine retrieval form
- capability to analyse any information in the EPR.

Although some clinical information would be available throughout an EPR's evolution (through the levels) in an adjacent data warehouse, the rich clinical detail required for systematic appraisal of clinical care, through clinical audit and clinical effectiveness, would be available once specialty or clinic-specific modules were developed. Examples of these are cancer modules or diabetes systems. These systems could be implemented at any time during the EPR's development but by level 5, all specialities would have their specific clinical data as a component of the EPR.

EPR level 6

This was the ultimate EPR level. Its characteristics were:

- telemedicine
- picture archiving communications systems.

Level 6 was conceived as the last stage of the evolution of clinical systems to support clinicians. It would include the development of the multimedia aspects including video, digital X-rays and photographs. However, it was always considered that a PACS could be implemented at any stage if a local business case could be produced. It is only in terms of the EPR that it followed the other components.

To help communicate the new ideas to the NHS, an interactive multimedia CD-ROM was produced as the final deliverable from the programme of work. It

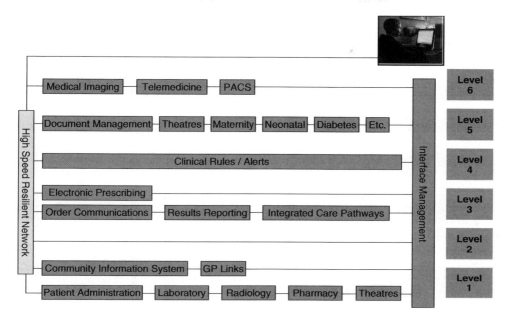

Figure 6.8 EPR levels with detail

contained a detailed description of each of the six EPR levels; with benefits anticipated from each level; a list of those suppliers who had products at each EPR level and sites currently in the NHS who had reached those levels of EPR. It also contained a vast assortment of papers and PowerPoint presentations which were of value to the Trusts embarking on this long journey.

The EPR programme did not identify what the passive record should contain or how it should be structured. It concluded that when treating a patient, all information and data formed the record, but the concept of 'active' and 'passive' EPR components emerged during the programme. This layered EPR model would later be picked up by *Information for Health* and used to set a target for the whole of the NHS (see below).

Through our trip down memory lane we have encountered a number of major initiatives with varying degrees of success. In order better to understand these elements and what now NPfIT must deliver through the NHS-CRS, it is of value to remember the three elements described above: integrated active clinical support systems; a passive record; and a data warehouse for secondary analysis.

The EPR programme was built around two core EPR Demonstrator Sites at Burton and Wirral. The programme also established a network of what were to become known as 'EPR Associated Sites' who undertook EPR developments at their own expense, but contributed to the general EPR learning. The programme also funded a number of individual EPR-related initiatives, one of which was to introduce a new paradigm to the approach to electronic records.

An orthopaedic surgeon, Mr Andrew Roberts, initiated a forward-thinking electronic records project, funded by the National EPR Programme, at the Robert Jones & Agnes Hunt Orthopaedic and District Hospital in Oswestry, close to the Shropshire/Wales border. It was forward-thinking because it adopted the use of SGML – Structured Generalised Mark-Up Language – as its architecture. SGML is an ancestor of XML, which has since become the communication standard for messages in all sectors including health. Without wishing to get into too much techie-talk, you will all know HTML – the formatting used in web pages. HTML tells the computer how to present the data within the web page: font, font size, colour, etc. SGML went one step further – it also described content and a degree of context to the words in the web page or web document, by attaching 'tags' to the text. So if you were writing a discharge letter, the SGML (or now XML) schema described not only how that document would appear but what structure the document should have: a tag would be attached to words that were describing patient's name or address. There may be a tag for 'presenting symptoms' and all the text following that heading would be tagged as 'presenting symptoms'.

This approach enabled retrospective searches through large text documents. It would allow, for example, a search for the term 'pain' within the context of presenting symptoms.

As we have since seen, some 10 years later, this approach is ideal for use in healthcare and does not restrict us to collecting structured clinical information solely through selection of rigid clinical terms. I digress, but it is helpful to understand this revolutionary piece of work which, at the time, was not widely welcomed by the traditional health informatics community.

Andrew Roberts went on to describe, in a characteristically clear way, the three different applications of clinical technology to the delivery of healthcare. He called them: Viewing, Doing and Chewing.

- 'Viewing' is the use of SGML/XML simply to view clinical information about a patient.
- 'Doing' is the adoption of integrated clinical systems which support the clinical care processes in real time (akin to the HISS applications and clinical work-station applications).
- 'Chewing' is the secondary analysis of information collected from the 'Doing' systems.

(The author proposes a fourth: 'Knowing' – making available to the clinician, electronic clinical knowledge and guidelines, at the point of care.)

Those three words charmingly describe the components of the EPR programme: the passive Electronic Patient Record and the Electronic Health Record – EHR (Viewing); the active EPR (including electronic orders, prescribing, Integrated Care Pathways) (Doing); and the data warehouse concept first introduced through the Resource Management Initiative (Chewing).

By this time then, we had all the evidence we needed to move this concept forward. A formal evaluation of the EPR programme was commissioned, and although some components of that evaluation were subsequently made public, the complete evaluation was never published.

In hindsight, this may have contributed to the lack of clarity which subsequently became apparent in the successor programme to EPR described below: ERDIP.

ERDIP

One of the strangest, and least understood, initiatives carried out by the NHS before NPfIT were the so-called 'ERDIP' pilots. Today it is hard to find anyone who can even remember what the acronym ERDIP stood for. It was, in fact, the NHS Information Authority's 'Electronic Record Development and Implementation Programme'.

ERDIP was an unfortunate acronym, and on reflection, a more appropriate title for the programme could have been Patient Record Implementation Development and Evaluation programme. On completion of the Electronic Patient Record Programme and following the publication of *Information for Health* (IfH), the ERDIP programme received the EPR baton. The EPR programme was passed on to a newly formed organisation – the NHS Information Authority (NHSIA) which had been formed as a result of the disbanding of the Information Management Group (IMG) of the NHS Executive.

The restructuring resulted in a policy component, which continued to be a part of the Department of Health – The Information Policy Unit; and a delivery arm, a Special Health Authority – the NHS Information Authority.

The NHS Information Authority established a programme of work taking forward the conclusions of the EPR programme as the Electronic Record Development and Implementation Programme – ERDIP.

ERDIP advertised for willing participants in a number of centrally funded projects which were advertised in two distinct categories: the EHR Demonstrators and the EPR Focus Groups. *Information for Health* suggested a number of beacon sites should be set up to explore the issues associated with the creation of EHRs. They would act as pathfinders to explore the development and implementation of EHRs and in particular the different approaches that could be adopted to achieve the EHR in practice.

It is worth reminding ourselves at this point that the EHR was the concept of a birth to death longitudinal record of care, fed by active integrated local organisational systems. It was the initial intention that the two distinct concepts of EPR and EHR as identified in IfH would be tested in a real environment. However, when these willing sites were selected, it became apparent that there was confusion as to the distinction between these two elements: EPR and EHR.

Projects which were obviously *EHR* in function were funded under the *EPR* Focus projects. This confusion is reflected in the final evaluation reports of PA Consulting when some of the sites (now all simply referred to as ERDIP EHR sites) expected EPR functionality (as defined in IfH) to be delivered through their EHR. At the same time, the more enlightened pilots sites had a clear appreciation that the EHR was fed by the local EPRs, which would have the 'active' functionality.

If a strategic decision was taken to morph these two concepts (EPR and EHR) together, there is no evidence for when this happened, and yet the result was that the two previously separate concepts – (1) active systems (EPR) and its passive record component and (2) the lifelong record (EHR) – were in fact amalgamated into the ERDIP EHR. This then became the Integrated Care Record Service (ICRS), and was eventually reincarnated as the National Care Record Service (NCRS), then the NHS-CRS.

As we will see when we look at the Government's *Information for Health* initiative later, the initial concept was of separate EPR and EHR elements: The

EHR was seen as a high level summary of an individual's clinical and social care record, which simply identified where additional information about a patient or citizen was stored. The EPR, on the other hand, was an integrated clinical support service producing a passive record component.

It was also the intention to deliver the local EPR systems first before attempting to deliver a national record for which there was no business case.

This is very confusing but it is important to raise these issues here, as there was intended to be a very clear distinction between the two concepts. That distinction seems now to have gone, and NHS-CRS as it is currently defined is attempting to be all these elements combined.

National evaluation of ERDIP sites

A National Evaluation of ERDIP sites[6] was undertaken by PA Consulting, who made the following recommendations and conclusions:

> The specification should set quantified targets of the benefits that 'ICRS access services' are required to deliver: this will require some further analysis and development work but will pay off in terms of clarity of objectives, drawing on the leading sites.
>
> A Knowledge Management website should be developed and used both to manage the programme, and to enable best practice to be identified and made readily accessible to all sites so they know both the standard to meet, and how to reach it.
>
> The provision of patient access to their own health records should best be addressed as part of the Health Record Infrastructure (HRI) work, not something that individual sites pursue.
>
> Change management aspects should be embedded within ICRS implementation plans and led by senior change management professionals supporting the StHA project directors, rather than by IT specialists.
>
> The NHS should ensure a higher standard of planning, budgeting and risk management than has generally occurred on the ERDIP programme.
>
> There are likely to be organisational change issues that should be managed and implemented at national level, supported by funding for organisational restructuring where applicable.
>
> To maximise the chance of success, future ICRS implementations should be run as fully funded projects with contractually defined deliverables.
>
> Conclusion: Clarity of definition of users, purpose, scope and performance is crucial in order to engage the stakeholders and ensure agreement across different care groups before commencing development. Where there is sufficient information to comment, all sites have shown the need for clarity of definition of users, purpose and scope. Indeed this step has proved crucial to engage the stakeholders and ensure agreement across different care groups *before* development commencing. North & Mid Hants, Cornwall, West Surrey, South & West Devon, Durham and Tees are just some of

those that exemplify the thorough approach needed. If not done thoroughly, with wide involvement of end users then it will prove much more difficult at later stages to ensure the EHR is incorporated into daily practice. West Surrey were thorough in other respects regarding required processes but did not agree performance criteria at the outset with their supplier, and as a result have procured a system that returns data in 2 to 5 minutes per enquiry.

There is also a lack of consensus around the processes that input (or create), update and use the EHR. Specifically, there is no consensus as to the relationship between [protocol-based referral], e-booking and e-prescribing processes.

ERDIP projects were generally successful in what they did and the comments made at the start of this section should not be construed as criticism of the individual projects or the efforts of those involved locally. The problem was the strategic significance of funding over 20 different projects which did not move the agenda forward proportionate to their efforts. In fact, their results may have caused more strategic confusion than clarification.

General conclusions of the National Projects/Programmes

What an intricate and convoluted history the story of NHS computing has been. We have seen waves of initiatives, white papers, pilots and strategies. Acronyms have been invented and discarded with abandon. Budgets have come and gone, organisational changes have rolled out, but the unwelcome reality remained as 2002 came around and the new National Programme was announced. Despite a generation of initiatives, the NHS remained stubbornly attached to its huge legacy of thousands of stand-alone systems from hundreds of different suppliers. Historically, national programmes and projects appear to have been managed with more effort and enthusiasm going into managing the project process and rather less time and effort devoted to the analysis of the outcomes. The attention has always seemed to be on ensuring that the deliverables were delivered as initially agreed, thus enabling a tick to be put in the box.

How could it all have been different? Well, before funding projects, it could have been made very clear what questions were being asked of the projects. It could have been clear that analysis of the outcomes should be planned. In the ERDIP case, for example, it looks as if there were no clear research hypotheses identified prior to identifying the pilots, and these appeared during the evaluation. This was apparent in the selection of *four* different EHR beacon sites of the ERDIP. If the purpose of the four EHR beacon sites was to identify a single model for the NHS, then a way to analyse and process the outcomes should have been in place at the time of contract award. But in the end, the confusion over what was EHR and what was EPR increased with the conclusion of the projects, and instead of clarifying this aspect of the programme, it resulted in the merging of the two concepts into what is now the NHS Care Records Service (NHS-CRS).

There is a generally held belief that ICT projects in the public sector are poorly evaluated. In a report by the Institute for Public Policy Research,[7] a leading progressive think tank, they acknowledge that eHealth is delivering benefit but just how much, they assert, is impossible to say because of a paucity of evidence.

They suggest that evaluations ensure that future projects are as successful as possible by allowing us to learn lessons from the past. Pilot projects should be allowed to fail if failure becomes inevitable. Failure is not, in itself, a negative outcome. A failure detected in a pilot project can reduce inappropriate investment and direction. However, the nervousness around computer projects generally – in government and healthcare specifically – results in a reluctance to publicly acknowledge a negative outcome from a project.

How else could it have been done better? The management of large IT projects in the past, in healthcare, has often been more about managing the project (did they deliver what they were funded to deliver?) rather than about an in-depth evaluation of the outcomes. In some circumstances, pilots were started without a clear idea as to why they were being funded at all, and pilots were sometimes a way of being seen to be active and delaying any fundamental strategic decision making.

That the complete formal EPR Programme Evaluation report was never published resulted in a lack of clear message as to its conclusions. ERDIP was very well evaluated, but the initial project foci were confused. That ICRS emerged as a merged EPR and EHR was apparently due to the NHS being unclear as to the difference between the two concepts. The handing of the EPR baton from the EPR programme to a new team of people (ERDIP) was not successful and may have created unnecessary confusion as to the vision.

Lessons learned

All the projects described concluded that the major factor to influence success of a project is the people and not the technology. In the HISS initiative, the same technology was often implemented at different sites with varying degrees of success. Those sites with positive support from clinicians succeeded more than those without. This was repeated in the Resource Management Initiative, where those sites using technology with strong clinical support and links to the Medical Audit initiatives had a more positive outcome than sites using identical technology that focussed purely on the management aspects of the programme.

Technology is just a tool which can only influence the outcome if the tool is used correctly and if it is used to redesign services. Professor Dennis Protti, who reported for the Information Policy Unit in 2002,[8] pointed out that over 150 factors had been identified as the key factors that can predict EPR/EHR implementation success, but only two are consistently associated with successful implementations. These two factors are top-management support and user involvement.

Several other factors were also repeatedly identified as influencing a positive outcome:

- Local champions who actively and enthusiastically promote the system, build support, overcome resistance and ensure the system is installed and used.
- Systems must be 'bedded in' for at least six months before decisions about the success of the technology can be made.
- Buy-in of the organisation is important. All users must see the need for change if they are to support it.

It seems that it is not technology that will make the programme a success, it is the people who will use this technology. Yes, the technology is important and it needs to be robust and easy to use, reliable and responsive. However, evidence shows that even relatively poor technology can, in the hands of enthusiasts, deliver real benefit to the clinicians and to the patients.

The two EPR Demonstrator Sites – Arrowe Park Hospital, Wirral and Queens Hospital, Burton – were both successful. Why? Did they get a load of central monies? No. They were virtually self-funded initiatives but they had considerable local clinical buy-in and the Chief Executive's support. Both hospitals organised, as one of their duties as EPR Demonstrator Sites, 'Open Days' where they showed the rest of the NHS how to do it.

Unfortunately not many others could follow in their footsteps. Why was that? It may have been lack of clinical commitment. More likely it was that fact that both Wirral and Burton had their EPR systems customised to fit around their work practices. That was possible as they were leading-edge and as national EPR Demonstrators the effort was considered worthwhile by their suppliers. But that would not be the case for those who followed. And herein lies another key message from the EPR programme. Local tailoring is essential and a one-size-fits-all solution will struggle to succeed.

It is also about willingness to change. Successful sites have used the opportunity offered by technology to rethink their care delivery. It is not just about having computers; in fact over the last 20 years there have been a considerable number of excellent projects which have delivered real benefits – even with the old ZX Spectrum or early BBC computers – because the enthusiasts have managed to coerce their colleagues to change their practices. Today we have all the technology at our disposal we should ever need. In fact, the pace of technological change makes it very difficult to stand still and implement when that implementation is already out of date. We are always chasing the rainbow. As soon as we get near to its end, it moves further away.

This isn't to say we shouldn't try. We may never get everyone using the very latest technology, because there will always be a lag time between emerging technologies and implementation. But even the successful implementation of relatively basic technology will radically change the delivery of healthcare forever.

The successful adoption of the new technology must require the desire or acceptance to change current working practices.

As Dennis Protti stated in his report for the Information Policy Unit in 2002,[8] 'Imagine a bunch of lumberjacks using chainsaws the same way they used handsaws by sawing back and forth. When the tools change, the people and business processes must adjust. Business value increases when users are determined to work with the new tools, but the value decreases when the users are not motivated.' So it is with clinical IT. It is a powerful tool to change and modernise the way NHS delivers care fit for this century, but the NHS must adjust.

Chapter 7

NHS IT policies and strategies

It often seems as if the NHS is in a continuous state of change. New policy documents and reorganisations are always with us, constantly changing the organisational structures that deliver the service. It is beyond the scope of this book to detail all the relevant policy documents, but in particular, the following have emphasised the role of information technology in the modern National Health Service. It is these policies that the National Programme for IT is expected to support.

- The NHS Plan[1]
- *e-Government Strategy*[2]
- *Shifting the Balance of Power.*[3]

And the technology strategies to underpin them:

- *Information for Health*[4]
- *Building the Information Core: Implementing the NHS Plan*[5]

The NHS Plan

The Government published their 10-year plan to reform the NHS in the year 2000. By any reckoning, it is an ambitious plan, which puts the patient at the centre of the NHS. You may have heard this term and may have dismissed it as political doublespeak. After all, the concept of patient-centred care was hardly new in 2000, and had been used for many decades before the NHS Plan was first published. But what is patient-centred care? And how is its delivery different to the NHS since 2000?

Kendall & Lissauer[6] identified five characteristics of patient-centred care:

- **It is safe and effective:** In other words, it is care that is intended to help patients; should not harm them; and interventions should be based on the latest evidence. This reinforces Hippocrates' mantra to 'at least do no harm'. It also reinforces the desire that only interventions that have previously had evidence of effectiveness should be considered. 'Common sense,' you may say. But analysis of current interventions and their outcomes often demonstrate that interventions are based more on local custom and are not always evidence-based. (There is also an issue as to what constitutes evidence, but this is not the book to discuss that.)
- **It promotes health and wellbeing:** Care should seek to prevent ill health and promote good health in addition to treating illness. Some say we currently have a National Illness Service, as our efforts to date have been focussed on treating ill people. However, the prevention of illness has as much, if not more,

of a role to play in any NHS. An example of this approach is the investment, by the NHS, in anti-smoking campaigns. Smoking currently costs the NHS billions of pounds each year.

- **It is integrated and seamless:** Holistic care must be based on people's social and emotional needs as well as their physical and medical ones and on a recognition that the individual's needs are linked to those of their family and community.

  Delivering a national health service that supports family and community needs *must* be planned and delivered as close to those communities and families as possible. That is not in Whitehall or in a Regional Office but at a level that can appreciate and evaluate those needs and put in place services that will satisfy them.

- **It is informing and empowering:** Patients should be provided with high-quality information to enable those who wish to become equal partners in decisions about their care to do so. It is one thing to suggest patients be empowered. It is quite another to provide those patients and citizens with the information with to make those choices. This is an essential part of patient-centred care.

- **It is timely and convenient:** It is important to patients that services are delivered in a timely and convenient manner and this also contributes to delivering better outcomes. The desire to move services to a more convenient location for the patient will have considerable implications for the NHS as it exists today.

The author, Michael Crichton, again in his book *Five Patients*, suggests that it was technology that defined hospitals in the last 20 years (this was written in 1970!), because as expensive, complex therapeutic and diagnostic equipment became available, the hospital assumed the role of providing a central location for such equipment. Today the cost of technology has been drastically reduced and the needs have changed. The NHS Plan describes a new service delivery model and technology provided through NPfIT will enable this patient-centric model to be delivered by moving more of this technology closer to the patient.

e-Government strategy

There was a time when it seemed as if every IT product, programme, or initiative had to be prefixed with an 'e' to make them appear more user-friendly. Even the government fell for this strange alphabetical fashion. The e-Envoy's Office (later to be renamed the e-Government Unit) announced in 2000 that all public services should be available online by the end of 2005. It was the launch of e-Government.

Perhaps this was a little ambitious. While the use of technology to reduce bureaucratic delays in an area renowned for it might have been a good thing, the desire to have *all* public services online seemed like IT for the sake of IT. However, the e-Government initiative has at least resulted in agreeing technical standards to enable this to happen, and the e-GIF Interoperability Framework document[7] cut through the waffle and firmly nailed its flag to a mast of standards that should be used for electronic communications in and between government.

The e-GIF defines the technical policies and specifications governing information flows across government and the public sector. They cover interconnectivity, data integration, e-services access and content management. The effect of this agreement at a national level is the acceptance of application and other standards in the heath sector such as XML and even at an application level. They even, for example, specify the use of Microsoft PowerPoint™ for presentations.

Shifting the balance of power

The Government's desire to refocus the NHS around the patient that we saw in the NHS Plan included the removal of several tiers of bureaucracy. These included the Regional Health Authorities, which were reduced from 13 down to 8 Regional Offices and then down to four regional directors of health and social care, and the 48 Health Authorities, which were reduced down to 28 Strategic Health Authorities. The reduction in tiers of management was intended to help put planning and spending as close to the local clinical community as possible. However, the most radical change was probably the emergence of Primary Care Trusts, who now have an increasing role as gatekeeper and commissioner of services.

Continuing technological developments will also enable the shift to delivering services at a local level. An example of this can be seen with the development of PACS – the ability to capture and store radiological images digitally. PACS enables the interpretation of an image to be made anywhere in the world. No longer will a patient *have* to go to a local hospital simply to have an X-ray. These images could be captured anywhere in the community. It could be done in a local diagnostic treatment centre or in a mobile radiological image lorry. And no longer does there have to be a trained radiologist on hand to interpret the image. The image can be transmitted anywhere for interpretation and opinion. It shows how the role of the hospitals will change as additional services begin to be delivered in the patient's local community.

NPfIT and the infrastructure it will deliver will be an enabler for this change.

Information for Health (IfH)

Of all the government policies that impacted healthcare IT, the one that remains at the centre was published in September 1998, predating the policies described above. It is considered here as the primary strategy document which underpins the National Programme for IT.

Information for Health was a Government white paper.[4] It followed on from the publication of the 1997 White Paper, *The New NHS: modern, dependable*.[8] Originally promised during the Healthcare Computing conference in March 1998 to be delivered 'while the daffodils are still in bloom', it was well worth the wait when it eventually appeared in September 1998, and was generally well received by NHS staff and the public. The crafty inclusion of a daffodil on the front cover made up for the slippage!

The approach adopted by the key author, Frank Burns, Chief Executive at Arrowe Park Hospital, Wirral, was to determine the information requirements of patients, healthcare professionals, healthcare managers and public. The applications required to deliver these information requirements were then identified and a pragmatic, incremental approach to delivery was identified, target dates set and a re-engineering process of the organisations to oversee the development and implementation begun.

Information for Health appears to have stood the test of time and many of the key elements identified in the strategy are the key elements of NPfIT. The principle adopted was to identify the requirement, identify the information objective, and finally to identify a portfolio of applications and services that would be required to deliver these objectives.

The strategic information objectives were:

- to ensure patients could be confident that the NHS professionals caring for them had reliable and rapid access, 24 hours a day, to the relevant personal information necessary to support their care
- to eliminate unnecessary travel and delay for patients by providing remote online access to services, specialists and care, wherever practicable
- to provide access for NHS patients to accredited, independent, multimedia background information and advice about their condition
- to provide every NHS professional with online access to the latest local guidance and national evidence on treatment, and the information they need to evaluate the effectiveness of their work and to support their professional development
- to ensure the availability of accurate information for managers and planners to support local Health Improvement Programmes and the National Framework for Assessing Performance
- to provide fast, convenient access for the public to accredited multimedia advice on lifestyle and health, and information to support public involvement in, and understanding of, local and national health service policy development.

The white paper suggested that, in order to ensure delivery of these strategic information objectives, the Government should require the NHS to achieve specific targets over a period of seven years. These targets were to be kept under review and developed in the light of changing needs and the capacity and availability of technology to meet them.

The specific targets were:

- reaching agreement with the professions on the security of electronic systems and networks carrying patient-identifiable clinical information
- developing and implementing a first generation of person-based Electronic Health Records, providing the basis of lifelong core clinical information with electronic transfer of patient records between GPs
- implementing comprehensive integrated clinical systems to support the joint needs of GPs and the extended primary care team, either in GP practices or in wider consortia (e.g. Primary Care Groups/Primary Care Trusts)
- ensuring that all acute hospitals have the ability to undertake patient administration, including booking for planned admissions, with an integrated patient index linked to departmental systems, and capable of supporting clinical orders, results reporting, prescribing and multi-professional care pathways
- connecting all computerised GP practices to NHSnet

- providing 24-hour emergency care access to relevant information from patient records
- using NHSnet for appointment booking, referrals, discharge information, radiology and laboratory requests and results in all parts of the country
- the development and implementation of a clear policy on standards in areas such as information management, data structures and contents, and telecommunications, with the backing and participation of all key stakeholders
- community prescribing with electronic links to GPs and the Prescription Pricing Authority
- routinely considering telemedicine and telecare options in all Health Improvement Programmes
- offering NHS Direct services to the whole population
- establishing local Health Informatics Services and producing costed local implementation strategies
- completing essential national infrastructure projects including the networking infrastructure, national applications, etc.
- opening a National electronic Library for Health with accredited clinical reference material on NHSnet accessible by all NHS organisations
- planning and delivering education and training in informatics for clinicians and managers.

EPR and EHR

As we saw when we looked earlier at the ERDIP pilots, the expressions 'electronic patient record' and 'electronic health record' (EPR and EHR) were terms often used to describe similar concepts. It may seem pedantic to dwell on this point, but labels can be important, and there is a clear distinction to be drawn here to define clearly how these terms were used in *Information for Health*.

Electronic Patient Record (EPR) was described as the record of the periodic care provided mainly by one institution. Typically this related to the healthcare provided to a patient by an acute hospital. EPRs would also be held by other healthcare providers, for example, specialist units or mental health NHS Trusts. It is also important to repeat that the record was expected to be the by-product of a set of integrated systems whose prime purpose was to support clinicians in the delivery of clinical care.

The term 'Electronic Health Record' (EHR), on the other hand, was used to describe the concept of a longitudinal record of patient's health and healthcare – from cradle to grave. It combined both the information about patient contacts with primary healthcare as well as subsets of information associated with the outcomes of periodic care held in the EPRs. For example, I would have one EHR but I would have several EPRs – wherever I had been treated.

The relationship between the two is illustrated below.

IfH envisaged that when a patient stayed in hospital, a subset of the information relating to that episode would form part of the EHR. What was not specifically made clear was that these organisational EPRs would have different facets:

- **The active components:** Including order communications; electronic prescribing and medicines administration; Integrated Care Pathways; specialist modules.

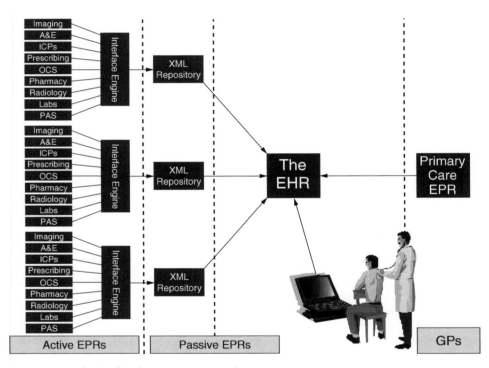

Figure 7.1 Relationship between EPRs and EHR

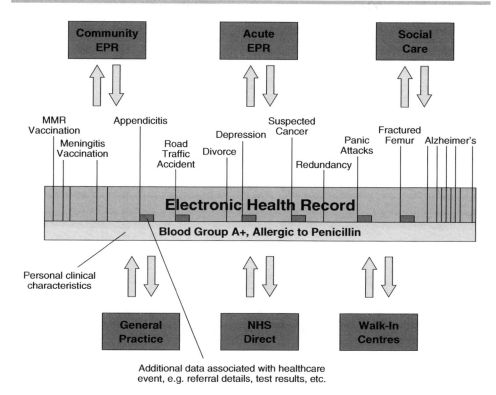

Figure 7.2 The Electronic Health Record

- **The passive components:** The output from the active systems is information and data which makes up the passive read-only electronic record.
- **Information for analysis:** Information for management monitoring and research would be derived from the active systems and made available for retrospective use in a data warehouse.

Information for Health also clarified the use of active systems to support long-term care, e.g. a mental health NHS Trust. The summary information would be passed on to the primary care team on a periodic basis to ensure that the EHR reflects the up-to-date status of the patient.

In certain circumstances, and with agreement of the appropriate professional and patient representative bodies, IfH went on to suggest that information from records held by social care organisations may also contribute to the EHR.

IfH concluded that, in theory, the EHR was therefore a combination of the bulk of the primary care EPR for a patient, together with linking information from other record systems for that patient. It did not propose a model for the EHR, but implied it would *not* exist until the organisational 'feeder' EPRs were in place.

Issues

Information for Health acknowledged that most of the NHS remains at the 'trailing edge' of information technology and several factors contributed to this.

Many GP systems (and community and mental health systems) that were currently in use at that time were proprietary systems with hardware and software which were incapable of coping with sophisticated EPR functionality. This, and the lack of a common primary care record structure, hampered the electronic transfer of records from one practice to another as patients change GP, the development of integrated primary/community care systems, and the ultimate development of an EHR.

The funding arrangements for GP information systems (partial reimbursement of the practice investment costs) perpetuate the problems encountered, and terms of service for GPs include a contractual commitment to keep paper records.

In many areas there was no active joint planning between hospitals and GPs of the messaging/communications technology needed to support the development of both hospital and primary care EPR.

The vast majority (>75%) of acute hospitals had yet to invest in the clinical information systems necessary to support EPR.

For community and mental healthcare there was a lack of agreement on what an EPR was and the development of systems had tended to be organisation-orientated and focused on administrative data.

In order to move this forward, IfH set targets for the NHS to achieve. The targets identified in the information strategy included:

- Over the period of this strategy all acute hospital sites would develop their information systems at least to the level necessary to support the new NHS target for clinical messaging with primary care, the wider strategic aims of this strategy, and internal EPR development. They should be able to support clinical activity such as placing clinical orders, results reporting, prescribing and multi-professional care pathways (i.e. to at least the level 3 functionality).
- By the end of 2002 all GP practices would be able to book some hospital appointments electronically.
- By the end of 2002, hospitals and all GPs would be routinely exchanging structured electronic messages for referrals, discharge summaries, laboratory and radiology requests/results.
- A specific national project would be established to advise on the circumstances for allowing remote out-of-hours access to Electronic Patient Records and the most practical options for securing this access.
- A number of sites would be identified as EHR beacon sites and would have developed plans by 2000 with a view to implementation by 2002.

Well, 2002 has been and gone. But don't be surprised that these same objectives, as outlined in *Information for Health*, are just as valid and, as you will see, are core to the aims and objectives of the National Programme for IT.

Data push or data pull?

IfH proposed that whether data collected during an episode was proactively dispatched to others caring for the patients (e.g. the GP) or whether the GP 'pulled down' data from a central repository were two not mutually exclusive options for the EHR/EPR model. It concluded that the result may be a hybrid solution where the majority of data is retained at the point at which it is generated – the hospital system in the example above – but messages containing a subset of that data are sent to the other system – the GP system. This subset may contain key items, e.g. a hospital discharge summary, to be integrated within the database of the GP system. Access to this locally held subset would be fast but there would also be a facility for the GP to retrieve the more detailed data from the hospital if required.

Making IT happen

When *Information for Health* was first published in 1998, the Information Management Group of the Management Executive of the Department of Health was the organisation charged with delivering information technology to the NHS. In addition to identifying the strategic direction of the development of ICT in the NHS, IfH also proposed an organisational restructuring to enable its delivery:

- The Information Management Group of the NHS Executive (IMG) would be disbanded and new national partnership arrangements for information introduced.
- Existing advisory machinery would be completely revamped to ensure there was an effective mechanism in place.
- Central policy making would be supported by an Information Policy Unit within the NHS Executive of the Department of Health.
- In order to allow the Regional Offices to deliver their key role in the partnership, work would be carried out to ensure that they have the skills and capacity necessary to undertake these functions. (Guess what? Regional Offices were disbanded as part of the 'Shifting the Balance of Power' reorganisation!)

Ensuring delivery of the national IM&T work programme to and for the NHS would become the responsibility of the NHS Information Authority, constituted as a Special Health Authority.

- The NHSIA would restrict its activities to those which could only be carried out nationally and would not take on any existing work that did not fully meet this criterion.
- The Family Health Service (FHS) Exeter Unit would be directly managed by the NHSIA, and a new specification for a replacement for the core Exeter computer system would be agreed with a view to procurement through a Public/Private Partnership. (The Exeter computer system was used by Health Authorities for maintaining GP lists, processing service payments, and call and recall systems.)

Addressing the procurement processes

A major overhaul of the existing IT procurement process was also identified as an area for immediate change. Because of the general nervousness about investing in IT, against a backdrop of IT failures, overly bureaucratic processes had been built into the IT procurement process. What was patently obvious was the number of levels of approval for relatively small investments – Health Authorities, NHS Executive Headquarters and Regional Offices. IfH reported that the Treasury had been involved in every information systems procurement with a capital cost over £1 million. This process was no longer tenable and had to be simplified. The requirements in *The New NHS* for NHS Trusts to clear major investments with their purchasers, coupled with the normal business case process, offered a way of establishing a more efficient approval process within new limits set to refer only the very largest procurements for Treasury approval.

National mandated processes for procurement

Information for Health suggested that the Government recognised the importance of ensuring widespread clinical 'ownership' of information, and in investing in clinical information systems. There was, however, a real concern to ensure that the local freedom to procure the technology necessary to deliver national information objectives did not result in needless local 'reinvention of wheels'. It suggested that this local freedom should not result in uneconomic, isolated, overambitious or poorly managed projects that failed to deliver the benefits to the clinical community.

Funding

Information for Health recognised the real difficulties in achieving the adequate funding of these ambitious IT projects.

It suggested that information technology must be regarded as a basic overhead cost for an organisation like the NHS, not as a novel or an unaffordable development. When NHS organisations consider that financing the IT infrastructure was necessary to deliver operational and strategic information needs, then it becomes a basic organisational need and therefore entirely different priorities will emerge.

> The NHS cannot afford not to make the investments necessary to deliver this strategy.
>
> Frank Burns

> My great concern is that any national solution would have to be watered down to make it nationally acceptable, and, for instance, they would drop out the prescribing component of any national EPR solution because the prescribing component is so culturally difficult. You have to work at this with the local community, so my worry would be the higher the level of centralization the lower the spec. So it would be a complete shell, a national e-mail system instead of what was intended.
>
> (Taken from interview with Frank Burns for *BJHC&IM* in 2002. *See* Appendix 1 for full transcript.)

Sir John Bourne (Head of the National Audit Office) found that the 1998 Strategy represented an improvement in design in several important respects. The inclusion of overall objectives provided greater coherence, and the development of agreed local implementation plans should also help. The NHS Executive expected new liaison arrangements to provide better communication about the Strategy in the NHS, and it intended to achieve better co-ordination than with the 1992 Strategy through a Programme Management Framework. The new Strategy included measures to increase the impact of specific projects, and the Executive also expected the evaluation work to be done within the NHS.

However, Sir John:

- considered that the Strategy's objectives and targets should be made specific and measurable if they are to be useful in monitoring expenditure and achievements
- was concerned that as with the 1992 Strategy, there is no overall business case, and he recommended that when business cases are produced for individual projects they address interdependencies between them and
- considered that there should be clearer plans for evaluation of the Strategy.

In the NHS it was generally accepted that *Information for Health* was a sensible, considered analytical review of the results of what has been piloted in the NHS over 20 years.

In describing the electronic records required to support the delivery of clinical care in a changing NHS, its distinction between the active systems (generally based within an organisation) and the recipient of summary information arising from those active systems was pragmatic. Why that proposed organisation-based EPR model was ultimately deemed inappropriate is discussed below.

The Integrated Care Records Service Initiative (ICRS)

And so we begin to unravel the most recent initiative. ICRS – which as a result of a name change became NCRS which then became the NHS-CRS – the core component of the National Programme for IT.

The 6-level EPR model we saw earlier, that emerged from the 3-year EPR programme, was a pragmatic and useful way of approaching the complex clinical IT issues, and was built on the previously described HISS initiative. However, the model was organisation-based, i.e. each hospital or Trust or GP practice had a separate and usually different EPR solution.

If the purpose of the EPR was simply to produce an electronic record then this would not cause a problem: each organisation could have been made to output the components of the electronic record in a standardised way.

If the purpose of the EPR was to collect clinical data for secondary analysis, these myriad solutions would not cause problems, as the analysis data outputted from these EPR solutions could have been standardised.

However, it was agreed that EPR was about supporting the delivery of clinical care, and the delivery of clinical care has been refocussed, putting the patient at the centre, rather than organising the delivery of healthcare around the organisations or health-carers. This would be impossible to deliver electronically if all the contributors to that care were in different organisations and therefore using different EPR systems. The ICRS initiative suggests that each organisation within a local community should use 'the same ICRS system'.

The National Programme for IT has gone further and suggests these local communities should be aggregated together into clusters or regions, and these clusters should have a single ICRS solution. This decision was not made solely in order to support the delivery of healthcare locally, but was also one of finance. Negotiating with suppliers for an EPR ICRS or NHS-CRS at a cluster level would deliver huge discounts as has been proven during this exciting and successful phase of the national programme.

The National Service Frameworks (NSFs)

Another reason to rethink the EPR model and its timetable emerged in 1999. This was because of the introduction of yet another new NHS strategy – the National Service Framework strategy. This was not an IT strategy, but it was clearly a strategy that would have IT implications. It was, put simply, a strategy that would focus on a small number of high profile diseases in an attempt to improve patient outcomes. Cancer, heart disease and diabetes are examples of the first NSFs. Targets would be set for GPs and hospitals for the treatment and processing of patients with these conditions. Each NSF has an associated information strategy – the Coronary Heart Disease Information Strategy,[9] for example, was published in 2001. It reinforced the assertion first voiced in IfH that the information collected to support care produces the data needed to carry out clinical audit as a by-product of care, not as an additional chore. It was expected that detailed specific clinical information associated with heart disease would be available as part of the level 3 EPR. But that was not expected to be implemented in all Trusts until 2005. Suddenly there was an example where the introduction of IT was lagging behind other NHS initiatives which needed it. Even if all Trusts had achieved the level 3 EPR by 2005, the specific specialist clinical information required to monitor NSFs was actually not in level 3 EPR but was anticipated to be available when the specialised systems were implemented at level 5. As a result, individual Trusts began to invest in (often) stand-alone clinical specialty systems, the sort we looked at in the last chapter, specifically to capture the clinical data for NSFs. This was a retrograde step and perceived (again) by the clinicians as a data collection exercise and of limited value to them in their day-to-day clinical role.

Building the Information Core: implementing the NHS Plan

This document considered the implications of the NHS Plan for the necessary information and IT infrastructure needed to support the patient-centred delivery of care and services.

It built on and updated *Information for Health*, the information strategy for the NHS, and provided a clearer focus on the priorities for successful delivery.

The document explained that whilst the e-government strategic framework required 'building services around citizens' choices', the NHS Plan required an 'NHS designed around the patient'.

In order to deliver these well co-ordinated 'seamless' services across 'whole systems', the information and IT systems needed to deliver these objectives must be capable of being personalised to meet the needs of the individuals who provide these services as well as those who receive them.

Information for Health had set out the strategic direction that supports both the NHS Plan and e-Government, and whilst much had been achieved in the two years since its launch, much still remained to be done and this document updated *Information for Health* in the light of the new policy agenda and developments in technology.

In order to achieve this, a number of new targets were set:

- **by March 2001:** 95% of GP practices and 25% of Trust clinical staff will have NHSnet connections and will be using NHS information services such as the National electronic Library for Health (NeLH)
- **by March 2002:** desktops will provide for NHS clinical staff basic e-mail, browsing and directory services, and the roll out of NHS cryptography support services begins
- **by March 2003:** migration to national standards for e-mail, browsing and office systems completed and all NHS staff with desktop access, and clinical information systems start to use the SNOMED Clinical Terms
- **by March 2004:** major national payroll/HR systems implemented
- **by 2005:** a vibrant networked NHS, with booking systems in place, electronic transfer of records within primary care, all acute Trusts with level 3 Electronic Patient Records and first generation Electronic Health Records.

In this section, we have revisited those policy documents which have set the scene for the National Programme for IT.

Targets have come and gone. Some have been hit, others missed.

The next section begins to unravel the IT requirements of these policy documents discussed above.

Chapter 8

Infrastructure

As Sir John Pattison remarked in his interview with the author in 2003 (for full interview *see* Appendix 2):

> The least 'exciting', but nonetheless fundamental to the success of all elements, is the work needed to put the infrastructure in place. The health service and the people who work in it and have cause to use it, should not have to 'make do' with inferior technology that other elements of society readily take for granted.
>
> We want to avoid giving those people less IT capability than their children receive at primary school, with high-speed networks now being made available to all schools and colleges. That means we should not have to accept a network that is slow and incapable of supporting the kind of fast data flows that clinicians will need. The infrastructure elements are essential building blocks to achieve the ultimate objective.
>
> Data and IT standards are essential if we are to allow flexibility in the delivery of clinical solutions. Interoperability between different components can only be achieved if dogmatic national technical standards are developed and complied with. The accreditation process will enable the implementation of these nationally agreed standards.

The next few chapters outline some of the key infrastructure elements on which the national programme for IT will be built.

Clinical coding

The NHS Executive stated in *Information for Health* that 'better care for patients and improved health for everyone depend on the availability of good information, accessible when and where it is needed'. But capturing clinical information in a structured way is not easy. Complex clinical conditions can be described in a variety of ways and often clinicians describe these conditions differently.

Imagine this problem. You want to review the outcomes of a group of patients with the same condition. But how can you identify the group if they are all described in different ways? The way around this clinical Tower of Babel is to introduce a common terminology – usually by implementing a systematic dictionary of clinical codes where every medical condition has a defined code. But even this has its difficulties. Just recording the fact that a patient is a smoker can use one of seven different codes. Stroke patients can be described by one of 50 or 60 different codes. Not a problem if you want to analyse data locally – you just find out what codes are used locally for the conditions you wish to study. But what happens if you want to look at, say, all the stroke patients in Yorkshire? Or in England? Are you beginning to see the problem?

It is essential to any health service that the interventions being used are successful. Monitoring at local, regional, national and international levels is essential if effectiveness of the delivery is to be maximised. The process is known as 'clinical audit'. It is a tool used as part of the clinical governance programme (clinical governance being a requirement for all organisations to be accountable for the quality of the delivery of care).

So, clinical coding is important, but again, not easy.

The collection of accurate and meaningful structured clinical data has generally been a process undertaken 'behind the scenes' by non-clinical coding staff with the resultant central returns (which contribute to the Hospital Episode Statistics (HES) data) having little clinical input.

The clinicians in the NHS have long suffered from a lack of routine clinical activity data and yet this is a prerequisite if a culture of continuing clinical evaluation and improvement is to be achieved.

Clinicians need good quality information for clinical audit, medical research and epidemiological studies. Health service manager need this information for budgeting, to assess the performance of health providers and for clinical governance.

Clinical information needs to be summarised to make it manageable, from the level of the individual patient up to national and international health statistics. This means that each piece of information needs to be encoded so that it can be analysed by computers. If clinical information is at the centre of the *Information for Health* strategy and therefore the National Programme for IT, then it is crucial that the NHS takes great care to adopt a good clinical coding system.

Hospital Episode Statistics (HES) provides information on admitted patient care delivered by NHS hospitals in England from 1989. This is used to provide wide-ranging analysis for the NHS, government and many other organisations and individuals who have an interest in health and healthcare administration.

HES covers all NHS Trusts in England but private hospitals are not included (although private patients treated in NHS hospitals are). The information can be used to answer a wide range of questions about topics such as:

- diagnoses
- operations (including day case surgery)
- Healthcare Resource Groups (HRGs)
- NHS Trusts
- Health Authority areas
- length of stay
- waiting time
- admission method
- patients' age, sex and ethnic group
- maternity care
- psychiatric care.

Read Codes

So we now know how important capturing clinical information in a meaningful and structured way is. So what has been done to date to help us achieve this?

A GP, Dr James Read, was a pioneer in the use of structured clinical information and in the 1980s he began to develop a system that would be known first as 'Read Codes' and later as Read Clinical Terms or 'Read CT'. Although Read Codes had their origins in primary care, they were developed with the medical and nursing professions as well as other Professions Allied to Medicine, to provide an agreed thesaurus of terms in everyday language for all healthcare professionals regardless of the setting.

It was envisaged that the extension of the application of the codes to all parts of the NHS would enable all clinical activity to be captured on computer. In 1987 the Joint Computing Group of the Royal College of General Practitioners and the General Medical Services Committee of the British Medical Association established a Technical Working Party to consider clinical classification systems for use in general practice. Its report, *The Classification of General Practice Data*,[1] published in August 1988, recommended that the Read Codes should become the standard way of recording medical data in general practice and that the implications of this should be considered throughout the NHS.

To facilitate the implementation of this report, the Read Codes were purchased by the Secretary of State for Health in 1990 and they became Crown Copyright. The Read Codes were endorsed in 1990 by the UK medical profession and by the NHS Management Executive as the standard clinical coding system in general practice.

The NHS recognised Read Codes as a source of primary coding in the Hospital and Community Health Services for the coding of diagnoses, operations and procedures, signs and symptoms and for all national minimum data sets and national statistics (central returns can be mapped from Read to other coding languages such as ICD-9 and OPCS-4 from mapping tables authorised for that purpose provided by the NHS Centre for Coding and Classification).

So what are these Read Codes?

The Read Codes are a comprehensive, hierarchically arranged, thesaurus of terms used in healthcare. Now that's a mouthful isn't it? This thesaurus has been coded, structured for use in computers, cross-referenced to important national and international classifications, and is dynamic.

The Read hierarchy

The Read thesaurus consists of a list of the preferred terms for each concept identified, organised into a hierarchy with increasing level of detail, and any number of synonyms (e.g. heart attack) linked to these preferred terms. An example of the five levels of detail found in the hierarchy follows:

> Level 1 Circulatory system diseases
> Read Code = G . . .
> Level 2 Ischaemic heart disease
> Read Code = G3 . . .
> Level 3 Acute myocardial infarction

Read Code = G30 . . .
Level 4 Acute anterior myocardial infarction
Read Code = G301 . . .
Level 5 Acute anteroseptal myocardial infarction
Read Code = G3011

Because the codes are hierarchical, analysis of the data can be achieved at the different degrees of detail. In the example above, a clinician could code one patient with acute anterior myocardial infarction. Another patient may be coded with *more* detail, so acute anteroseptal myocardial infarction, or *less* detail, simply acute myocardial infarction. But because the codes are hierarchical, analysis can be performed at level 3 (acute myocardial infarction), which would include all three examples described above.

Unlike other classifications in use in primary care and elsewhere, the Read Codes had been developed specifically for use with computers. Their structure within computer systems allowed for terms to be found using natural language without the need to understand, remember, or even see the codes themselves. This was a major advance for clinical coding. The Read Codes were at least as detailed as, can be mapped to, and are compatible with, other widely used standard statistical national and international classifications, such as ICD-9, ICD-9-CM and OPCS-4.

But if there is already a coding scheme – International Classification of Disease (ICD), why did the NHS need Read? There's a clue in the name. ICD is international. This means it requires agreement from the international community before new codes can be released. Understandably that could take years, and in fact ICD codes are updated generally every 10 years. If we want clinicians to describe what they are doing in a way that is meaningful to them, we can't restrict their descriptions with codes that could be 10 years out of date. And ICD is a coding system – not a terming system. We want doctors to describe what they've done in clinical terms or words. ICD is not sufficiently clinician-friendly, and would not appear in a clinician-friendly way in the electronic record.

Read Codes or any clinical terming process must map to ICD to enable international comparisons of data to be achieved. The mappings enable the data captured locally to be analysed nationally or even internationally, if desired.

Clinical terms

Read Codes evolved from what was known as the original '4-Byte Set' where each code consisted of only four alphanumeric characters. This grew into the 5-Byte Version 1, which was developed to include specific functions for cross-references to central returns for hospitals, as well as providing functionality for GPs. In this version, Read Codes were extended to five alphanumeric characters, allowing a five-level hierarchy, with text descriptions of up to 30 characters.

In 5-Byte Version 2, the codes were identical to 5-Byte Version 1, but text descriptions were extended to include 60- and 198-character versions.

The dynamic quality of the Read Codes (where new codes can be added if required) is essential if healthcare providers are to use computerised patient record systems, because the practice of medicine is constantly changing. New concepts and procedures evolve, as do new drugs and therapeutic agents, and these have to be represented in the Read Codes immediately so that clinicians and other users can take full advantage of these systems and record accurately what they are doing.

But there were problems with the strict hierarchical structure. There were occasions, for example when a clinical condition like *Tuberculosis meningitis* could be positioned in different hierarchies. In this instance, *Tuberculosis meningitis* could be placed in the Infectious Disease chapter *and* in Nervous System and Sense Organ Disease. How would you know which code to search for if you wanted to find all patients with *Tuberculosis meningitis*?

There were other problems with only five levels of detail and when a more descriptive text was required, problems were encountered. In order to overcome these problems, a complex and comprehensive programme of work was started. It was called the Clinical Terms Project (CTV3), and it was developed to address the problems of the early versions as described above. Clinical terms replaced the old Read Codes as the method for capturing structured clinical and social information. The terms had a completely redesigned architecture which consisted of terms, concepts, and descriptions which enabled greater degrees of flexibility in how to assign a structure to a fluid clinical language.

It is beyond the scope of this book to go into detail on complex clinical coding. Suffice it to say that the strict hierarchy was replaced with a more flexible structure, where the hierarchy is formed by a set of 'parent–child' links held in this file, rather than being code-dependent. Any 'parent' can have several children, and a 'child' can have several parents.

The final stage of Read Codes evolution was the incorporation of Clinical Terms V3 into the American Pathologists SNOMED thesaurus to become SNOMED CT.

SNOMED CT

The name SNOMED is an acronym, of a sort. It stands for 'Standard Nomenclature of Medicine', and it aims to be just that, an exhaustive catalogue of medical terms. For over 40 years the College of American Pathologists has invested in the research and development of SNOMED. It has successfully moved from its early origins as a pathology-centric terminology (SNOP), to SNOMED II and SNOMED III, nomenclatures that cross medical specialties used in clinical computer applications.

In collaboration with the Kaiser Permanente organisation since 1995, the College revolutionised the structure of SNOMED to reflect the advances in medical informatics and the science of computing resulting in the SNOMED Reference Terminology (SNOMED RT) that was launched in May 2000.

At this point there could have been a conflict between the growing use of Read Codes in the NHS, and the gradual international acceptance of SNOMED. But unexpectedly, a pleasant compromise was achieved. To achieve world class terminology status and conserve the limited global supply of medical terminology expertise, the American College of Pathologists, owners of SNOMED, and the UK's Minister of Health agreed to combine SNOMED RT with the UK's Clinical Terms Version 3 (formerly known as the Read Codes) to create what is now known as SNOMED Clinical Terms (SNOMED CT). SNOMED CT, first released in January 2002, combined the strength of SNOMED RT in the basic sciences, laboratory and specialty medicine, including pathology, with the richness of the

UK's work in primary and secondary care. The end result is a comprehensive and precise clinical reference terminology that provides unsurpassed clinical content and expressivity for clinical documentation and reporting.

The final piece in this complex and critical jigsaw is the Health Language application. This sits within a clinical application and manages the updates from SNOMED CT. Whichever coding system is used, clinicians should not need to know it as they interface with the clinical application and automatically collect clinical terms by the use of their own words. The Health Language module coupled directly to the terms does the rest.

Potential of clinical coding

We have seen the development of the capture of structured clinical terminology to SNOMED CT, but how important is this to NPfIT? How will these comprehensive terms be applied and bring benefit?

One of the major purposes of collecting structured clinical data through clinical coding should be to enable clinicians in primary and secondary care settings to monitor the effectiveness and efficacy of the care being delivered. At present in most hospital trusts in the NHS, clinical coding is restricted to inpatient and day cases only (with some outpatient operative procedures being reported). If the purpose of collecting clinical information is to support the clinical governance agenda and to contribute to the efficient management of clinical resources, then inpatient data in isolation is of limited value.

Collecting clinical information in outpatient clinics is essential and will eventually become a mandated requirement. In addition, the real-time use of clinical codes during the delivery of clinical care (through clinical decision support tools, monitoring adverse events and linking patients to Integrated Care Pathways) will demand outpatient coding in real-time.

Adverse event tracking

While coding has a role in recording clinical activity for retrospective purposes, it has a far greater potential in the real-time support of the delivery of clinical care. In a US paper entitled 'Detecting adverse events using information technology'[2] Bates *et al.* report:

> . . . developing and maintaining a computerised screening system generally involves several steps. The first and most challenging step is to collect patient data in electronic form. The second step is to apply queries, rules, or algorithms to the data to find cases with data that are consistent with an adverse event. The third step is to determine the predictive value of the queries, usually by manual review.
>
> The data source most often applied to patient safety work is the administrative coding of diagnoses and procedures, usually in the form of ICD-9-CM and CPT codes. This coding represents one of the few ubiquitous sources of clinically relevant data. The usefulness of this coding – if it is accurate and timely – is clear. The codes provide direct and indirect evidence of the clinical state of the patient, co morbidity, and the progress of the patient during the hospitalisation or visit. For example, administrative data has been used to screen for complications

that occur during the course of hospitalisation. However, because administrative coding is generated for contract monitoring and legal documentation rather than for clinical care, its accuracy and appropriateness for clinical studies are variable at best. The coding suffers from errors, lack of temporal information, and lack of clinical content. Coding is usually done after discharge or completion of the visit; thus its use in real-time intervention is limited.

(So these coding problems are encountered in America too!)

Bates continues:

> despite these limitations, administrative data are useful in detecting adverse events. Such events may often be inferred from conflicts in the record. For example, a patient whose primary discharge diagnosis is myocardial infarction but whose admission diagnosis is not related to cardiac disease (e.g. urinary tract infection) may have suffered an adverse event.

The role of the clinical codes in the real-time delivery of clinical care will require a new model for its collection and one which will require live coding during the episode, rather than retrospectively as present.

Decision support

If clinical codes were assigned during an episode, these will become the 'trigger' with which to activate decision support tools. As an example, if a patient is suspected of having a myocardial infarction (MI), the code could activate a 'to do' list for suspected MIs or a 'recommended investigations' profile.

Clinical terms and their underlying codes will also determine the way that a patient is assigned to an Integrated Care Pathway which will, in turn, ensure conformance to a locally agreed plan or pathway for treating specific conditions.

The future of coding

While it is impossible to predict the future of coding, we can make some speculations based on the past and knowing what is likely to happen in the future in terms of technology development. Regardless of the evolution of classification of clinical data, it is clear that the need for this data – and more of it – is likely to increase. We have become an information-driven society. As such, the ability to turn diseases, symptoms, treatments (in the form of procedures), exposures and causes into data that can be analysed in aggregate is attractive to many – including providers, the government, researchers, pharmaceutical companies, insurance companies, vendors to the healthcare industry, employers and consumers of healthcare. This list covers just about everyone.

Although the demand for the work of a clinical coder is likely to increase, the methodology used by that coder is likely to evolve into a more efficient process – one that is rich in technology as well as intellectual capital. After all, would the coder of 1960 have ever imagined that her beloved coding book would be replaced by a computerised encoder? Not likely. The important point to make here is that the coder as the manager of the process of coding did not disappear when the coding book gave way to the encoder. Rather, the coder needed to develop an entirely new set of skills focused on computer technology. In the future, it is likely that technology will play an ever increasing role in documentation and coding and classification systems, and NPfIT has acknowledged the importance of this clinical coding and is central to the solutions being implemented through the NPfIT contracts.

The new NHS number

If we aim to bring clinical and other information about a patient together in one place, we need to be absolutely sure that all the information about that individual patient has been correctly and completely 'captured and assembled'. We must be confident that every patient on the system is uniquely and accurately identified. In order that all these disparate data items, scattered around the country, are able to be assembled in a single patient's file, each data item needs to have a unique identifying number. In this case, the NHS number.

The NHS number is not new, although this latest version is so described. The need to introduce an NHS number for all patients came as a result of the National Health Service Act, which came into force on 5 July 1948. Under the Act doctors were paid per capita for all persons registered with them, so it became important to keep track of patient movements, their deaths, details of when they happened to enlist in HM Forces or when they chose to leave the United Kingdom. To achieve this, it was essential that each patient had a unique identifying number.

From 1950s until the issue of the *new* NHS number in 1996, the NHS number was used as a means of communication between the National Health Service Central Register (NHSCR), the Executive Councils and all NHS organisations to facilitate the timely and accurate transfer of medical records and had virtually no other purpose save local arrangements. The use of the NHS number today, the *new* NHS number, allows patient data to be assembled in one place regardless of where that data has been derived. It allows electronic access to patient details via secure online access, resulting in better communication with patients, and this in turn helps to improve medical care by reducing the amount of out of date or inaccurate patient data held.

The new style of number was introduced in 1996 in England and Wales, replacing a variety of inconsistent predecessors. The first nine numbers are the identifier and the tenth is a check digit used to confirm the number's validity.

Patients are given their unique identifier when they 'join' the NHS either by approaching an NHS GP surgery or health centre for the first time and asking to permanently join their practice list, or by approaching a Health Authority, who will allocate them to a local NHS GP practice list.

Babies born in England and Wales are now allocated an NHS number soon after birth by Maternity Units at the point of Statutory Birth Notification.

The NHS Strategic Tracing Service

The NHS Strategic Tracing Service is a national (England and Wales) database of people, places and NHS organisations. It sits at the heart of the modern healthcare agenda as a vital tool for sharing information within the National Health Service. NHS staff can, subject to security procedures, use the Tracing Service to access their patient's demographic details – usually their name, address, date of birth, GP name and address details. They can obtain the NHS number too, and a range of up-to-date administrative information.

The NHS-Wide Clearing Service

The NHS-Wide Clearing Service (NWCS) provides a means of exchanging and processing high volumes of data between NHS user organisations through its three core functions. Thus NWCS:

- facilitates the flow of data from (Hospital) Trusts and Primary Care Trust (PCT) Providers to all Primary Care Trusts to support commissioning
- facilitates the flow of data from Trusts and PCTs to Department of Health to support national performance management and strategic service planning
- provides strictly controlled access to its database for approved organisations for individually specified purposes.

NPfIT's Secondary Uses Service will take the data flowing from the NWCS and over time enrich this data from additional data sources.

Chapter 9

The shape of the fog

It is time to zoom out now on this great national programme to try and get a view of the shape and dynamics of this enormous project. Earlier I described NPfIT as a city draped in a fog – where close-up the buildings are perfectly clear, but from a distance there seems to be very little shape or structure. Zooming out, with the benefit of a map, we can see some shape in the fog.

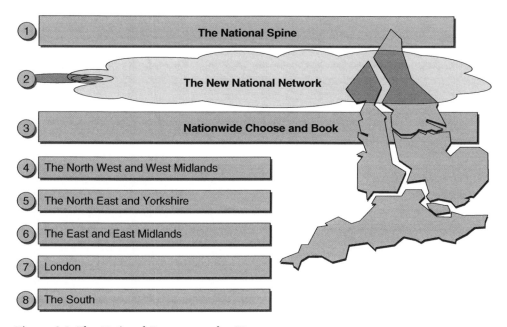

Figure 9.1 The National Programme for IT

Delivering NPfIT: NISPs, NASPs and LSPs

Three groups of providers have been defined as part of NPfIT. All three will work closely together to deliver integrated services.

National Infrastructure Service Providers (NISPs) will deliver infrastructure components nationally.

National Application Service Providers (NASPs) will deliver national applications. Local Service Providers (LSPs) will be responsible for delivering the local aspects of the NHS-CRS.

National Infrastructure Service Providers (NISPs)

The provision of national infrastructure to underpin the services and applications provided nationally and locally, will be delivered by what are known as NISPs – National Infrastructure Service Providers.

An example of such a service is the provision of broadband network across the NHS. As described earlier, the New NHS National Network (or N3) will be a service provided by BT acting as a NISP.

National Application Service Providers (NASPs)

Any application which is required as a national resource, in contrast to the applications being delivered locally in clusters by the LSP, will be provided by a National Applications Service Provider e.g. the NHS-CRS data spine component will be delivered by BT acting as a NASP.

Local Service Providers (LSPs)

For contracting purposes, the Department of Health divided the country into five 'clusters' of strategic health authorities and ran competitions in each to select a dedicated Local Service Provider (LSP).

These five clusters, described in detail later in the book, are:

- Eastern
- London
- North East
- North West and West Midlands
- Southern.

Each Strategic Health Authority has a Chief Information Officer (CIO) and each has a key role in ensuring Primary Care Trusts (PCTs) and NHS Trusts implement and use the core IT solutions determined at national level. The LSP will work with each strategic health authority to integrate, and where necessary replace, existing IT infrastructure to meet the needs of the national programme. Initially each will deliver a full range of ICRS, and an IT help desk service to provide a single point of contact for all users.

What will they deliver?

NHS-CRS: the national data spine

The National Care Records Service is the core service in the programme. It will bring a number of benefits to the NHS including access to integrated patient data, prescription ordering, proactive decision support and best practice reference data.

Phase one of the NHS-CRS specification, which is to be delivered by December 2004, states that all clinicians should be able to browse Internet/intranet sites and view basic clinical information about their patients online. At this time one

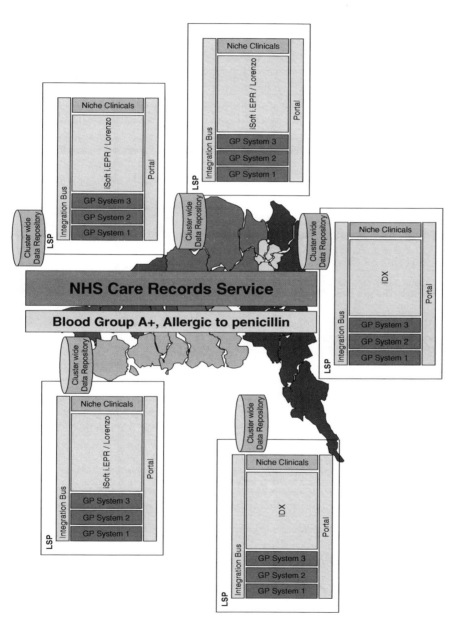

Figure 9.2 Local NHS-CRS and the data spine

third of hospitals will support electronic X-rays. Phase two will give clinicians access to a more comprehensive patient record including specialist results, GP prescribing history, hospital discharge summaries and clinical documentation. Future phases up to 2008 will deliver comprehensive, community-wide patient records with support for care pathways and appointment scheduling across different NHS organisations as well as inpatient and outpatient prescribing in hospitals.

The spine is not simply a repository for clinical information but is also an active component of any transactions undertaken locally. Yes, the spine will control who has access to which patients' clinical information but it will also be the gatekeeper to any local clinical functionality delivered through the LSP's NHS-CRS service. Nothing can be done in any local LSP without the user going through an authentication process within the spine.

The spine also maintains the patients' 'demographic' data – keeps the personal information about every member of the population up to date; address; registered GP, change of names etc. as previously described in the NHS Strategic Tracing Service.

Electronic transfer of prescriptions (ETP)

In September 2003 electronic transfer of prescriptions (ETP) was also added to the specification for NHS-CRS. ETP will reduce some of the administrative burden in managing repeat prescribing. Much more crucially, feedback from the pharmacies will enable clinicians to know if patients are collecting their medications. In certain cases, GPs will be able to devolve the routine management of repeat prescriptions to community pharmacists. At present, the paper prescription, completed and signed by the GP, cashed/dispensed by the community pharmacist, ultimately ends up in the Prescribing Pricing Authority (PPA) in Newcastle where the handwritten data is manually input into the PPA database. This provides useful medication information to be fed back to local GPs and Primary Care Trusts.

Finally, the electronic transmission of prescriptions will enable monitoring of entitlement to free medications to be undertaken which will have the potential to reduce fraud by up to £3 billion per annum.

How does ETP work?

At present, a patient will go to her GP and, more often than not, leave with a paper prescription. The patient can go to any chemist to 'cash' the prescription and that chemist may, or may not, keep a record of the patient's prescription on a computer. However, if a patient does not always go to the same chemist, there is no one place where that patient's complete medication record is held.

In the ETP pilots, a number of models were tested: The patient can nominate their dispensing chemist of choice. In this case, the prescription (generated by the GP's patient record system) would be sent electronically to the nominated chemist, and a copy be transmitted to the patient's electronic record. The patient would later collect the drugs, or could have previously arranged to have the drugs sent to their home.

In the second model, where the patient did not have a nominated chemist for dispensing, the patient would be given a printed 'token' and the electronic

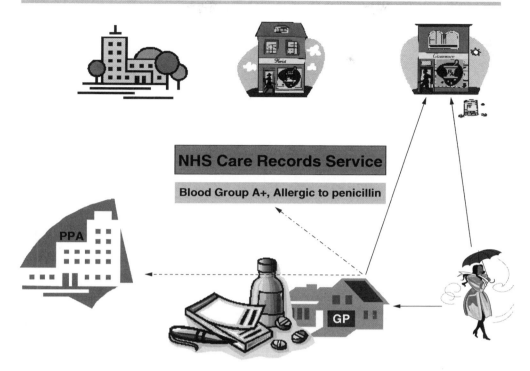

Figure 9.3 The ETP Model 1: patient selects chemist

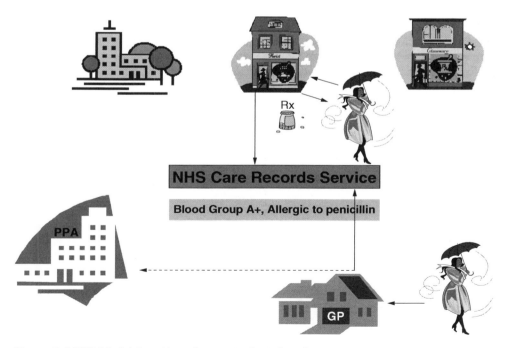

Figure 9.4 ETP Model 2: patient does not select chemist

prescription would be held centrally as part of the patient's electronic record, and only when the patient presents at the chemist with their printed token would the pharmacist retrieve the prescription and dispense it.

In both cases, copies of all electronic prescriptions would be automatically transmitted to the Prescriptions Pricing Authority for their use in managing payments and reimbursements.

The electronic transmission of prescriptions component of the programme was subsequently included in NHS-CRS functionality and not as a separate project.

Choose and Book

The e-booking system will operate across the NHS and is intended to give patients more choice and control over their hospital appointments. GPs and other clinicians will also be able to book patient appointments and consultations immediately rather than waiting for an appointment letter.

The NHS Choose and Book website (*see* Appendix 4) describes the service as, 'A national service that will, for the first time, combine electronic booking and a choice of time, date and place for first outpatient appointment. By the end of 2005 it will be available to all patients in England requiring elective care (over 10 million each year).'

Choose and Book will enable patients to choose a convenient place, date and time for their initial hospital appointment. By the end of 2005, patients in England will be able to choose from one of four or five hospitals (or other healthcare provider facilities) commissioned by their PCT. Information on these hospitals will be provided to GP staff and patients at www.nhs.uk to enable them to choose.

Patients can either book their appointment electronically immediately with the GP or other practice staff, or they can call a telephone booking service or use the Internet at a later stage.

This is a big step in giving patients greater involvement in the choices and decisions about their treatment.

This initiative is not without its problems, not only technical where linking multiple and different electronic diary components of the hospital Patient Administration Systems is a prerequisite, but also organisation challenges.

At present, the specialist is the one who can assess the requirements of multiple patients referred by different GPs and assign a priority to their case.

With direct booking of outpatient appointments, who is to say that patient Jimmy Rawthorpe from GP X requires a quicker appointment than patient Norah Jones from GP Y?

There is a degree of nervousness from both GPs and hospital consultants with this part of the national programme, nerves which may be placated with the adoption of clinical decision support rules being built into the referral pathway.

This will reduce inappropriate referrals, which may be considerable, and ensure consistency of prioritisation.

'Patient choice' is a key political objective, although in reality evidence shows that the majority of patients would prefer to continue to be treated by their local hospital.

The New NHS Network (N3)

As discussed in the previous section on infrastructure, a rapid, secure, robust and reliable network is an essential component of the national programme, without which the national implementation of clinical IT will not happen.

This network must be robust and have enough capacity (bandwidth) to enable rapid and efficient communication within and between NHS participants.

The implementation model proposed for NPfIT, with large cluster data centres hosting the cluster applications and the requirement to manage access control centrally (on the data spine) is totally dependent on an efficient, rapid network.

Historically, however, the NHS network has been an Achilles heel, the weak point in the IT infrastructure of the service. It has been criticised for being too slow, too insecure and too open to failures. N3 is the name for the New NHS Network that will aim to address these concerns by providing wide area networking services to the NHS in England. N3 will provide substantially increased bandwidth over the current NHSnet and greater value for money. It will enable the implementation of the NHS Care Records Service, the Electronic Booking Service and the Electronic Transmission of Prescriptions Service.

All N3 services will be provided to the NHS by the N3 Service Provider. This is regardless of any service that might be sourced from third parties or sub-contractor organisations.

N3 services are specified to provide ample wide area network connectivity to support site-wide Internet and e-mail access and the implementation of NPfIT applications. The N3 services are more advanced and complex than the current NHSnet services. In particular, the high availability figures and segregation of data based upon quality of service mapping signal a move away from concentrating on absolute bandwidth.

NHS-CRS: local solutions

As we will see later in this book, it is the active components of what is collectively known as the NHS-CRS which will deliver the greatest clinical benefit. Yes, a shareable electronic record will also give benefit, but the *real* clinical benefit is the implementation of electronic prescribing, electronic order communications, Integrated Care Pathways and ultimately telemedicine – remote home care support. All these components, when coupled to clinical decision support tools, have the capacity to radically improve the effectiveness of clinical care.

These NHS-CRS components will be discussed in greater depth later in the book.

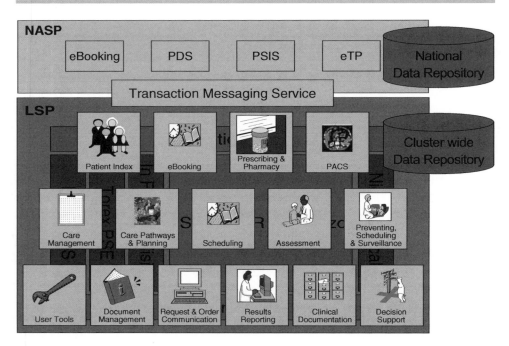

Figure 9.5 Local NHS-CRS functionality

Chapter 10

The NHS-CRS clusters

Back when the National Programme for IT was in its early stages of development, in the early months of 2003, there was much discussion about the geography that would descend upon the new computerised NHS. Sir John Pattison had spoken about 'four or five' service providers – but somehow the expectation was that the NHS would be carved up and offered out to competition in small, discrete parcels. The favourite suggestion was that there would be 28 medium-sized procurements – one for each Strategic Health Authority. The NHS would become a mosaic of different computer systems, shared out among half a dozen or so service providers.

It wasn't to be. When the invitations finally went out to the competing suppliers, a whole new set of geographic boundaries had been drawn onto the map of England. The NPfIT will be delivered via organisational structures called clusters that we first met in the opening chapter of this book. Five clusters have been established for the NHS in England:

- Eastern
- London
- North East
- North West and West Midlands
- Southern.

These are curious entities, these clusters. They have no real existence, except as bureaucratic lines on a map. Until NPfIT they had no offices, no staff, no budgets, no power to award contracts. They are a loose, almost random, coalition of SHAs. Another group at another time might have drawn the lines differently. No matter. The contracts would be let by the NHS and administered centrally.

So each cluster consists of a conglomerate of between four and seven Strategic Health Authorities (SHAs) and their constituent Trusts and organisations working together to govern, manage and implement the programme.

Local health communities will themselves take responsibility for implementation of the Programme. As statutory bodies SHAs and their constituent organisations have responsibility for the planning, development, implementation and where necessary resourcing of the NPfIT.

The cluster acts as a facilitative and co-ordinating body across its geographical area and supports local processes and procedures on an advisory, contract and service management level. Additionally clusters provide support and expertise on the business benefits of the programme and the stakeholder and communication aspects of the programme.

Each cluster has a Regional Implementation Director (RID) who led the input to LSP negotiations and is leading the implementation process across the cluster. The

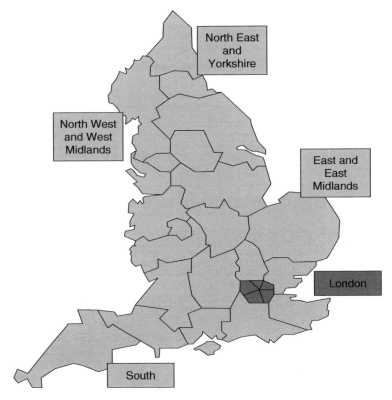

Figure 10.1 The clusters

RID manages the programme support team and the relationship with local supplier, as well as co-ordinating deployment.

Each group of SHAs has created a programme board for their cluster and nominated a lead Chief Executive Officer to chair it. All SHA CEOs sit on the board, together with their Chief Information Officers, stakeholders from across the cluster area and members of the National Programme Team. The role of the board is to provide senior management level endorsement for the rationale and objectives of the local programme, promote and support the changes introduced, and champion the new functionalities to be delivered. It is also tasked to ensure that benefits and desired outcomes are achieved and to arbitrate on any disagreements that may occur within the cluster.

Each cluster also has a programme management group (PMG), also known as Cluster Programme Boards in some clusters, which are made up of CIOs and programme managers from every SHA area, plus the RID and key members of the cluster support team, and LSP representatives. The PMG will co-ordinate and manage the progress of the National Programme across the cluster, dealing with issues such as progress monitoring, issue resolution, risk management, planning, sharing good practice and deployment of resources.

SHA CIOs are responsible for the implementation of solutions and the delivery of benefits at an organisational level across the SHA, reporting to the PMG on progress and issues, and receiving leadership, guidance and support from their RID and programme support team.

Similar programme management structures are in place to take forward National Programme implementation within each SHA. A programme board and programme team has been set up, with project teams working on each of the key deliverables within the overall programme.

Work is well advanced in clusters and local organisations to draw up plans for programme implementation in conjunction with the relevant Local Service Provider and to quantify and identify the resources required, both physical and financial, to support the phased deployment, implementation and realisation of the NPfIT.

Staff from the clusters and the central NPfIT team will work with LSPs and NASPs to ensure that they are engaging NHS staff appropriately in implementation planning and system delivery.

The North West and West Midlands cluster

The North West and West Midlands cluster (often affectionately called the 'M6 cluster' because of the way that the M6 motorway serves the whole area) stretches from Carlisle and Workington in the north to Hereford in the South.

It includes the major cities of Liverpool, Manchester and Birmingham as well as town and cities as diverse as Coventry, Dudley, Shrewsbury, Chester, Stoke, Bury, Blackburn, Preston, Lancaster, and Barrow in Furness – among others.

This is the cluster with the second largest population, but the largest current NHS IT spending. It has an impressive track record; Burton and Wirral Hospitals were among the early HISS sites, and were two of the three NHS Demonstrator Sites for Hospital EPR. Salford Hospital and University Hospital Birmingham use iSOFT Clinical Manager. Walsall and South Staffordshire communities led a very successful ERDIP project in the development of community wide records and South Warwickshire PCT is leading on a National Programme for Information Technology demonstrator for primary care systems.

The CSC Alliance

The Local Service Provider (LSP) for the North West and West Midlands is an alliance of companies led by Computer Sciences Corporation – CSC.

CSC is a global IT services company, with headquarters in El Segundo, California. They employ 90 000 people worldwide, and in 2004 they had a global turnover of $14.8 billion. They have over 8000 people in the UK, and their key strengths include their huge outsourcing capability and their systems integration expertise.

CSC has a record of bidding successfully for huge public IT projects. In 2003 they won a project with the Royal Mail which compares favourably in size with their task in the North West and West Midlands.

For the National Programme for IT, CSC has formed an alliance with a number of critical partners. Their main solutions partner is iSOFT, a Manchester-based company that we first encountered in this book as a supplier of Resource Management systems. We will learn more about iSOFT later on. Along with iSOFT, the US technology giant SCC joins CSC Alliance as the key technology

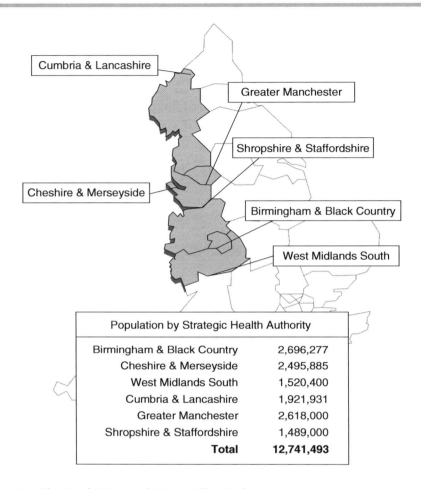

Population by Strategic Health Authority	
Birmingham & Black Country	2,696,277
Cheshire & Merseyside	2,495,885
West Midlands South	1,520,400
Cumbria & Lancashire	1,921,931
Greater Manchester	2,618,000
Shropshire & Staffordshire	1,489,000
Total	**12,741,493**

Figure 10.2 The North West and West Midlands cluster

provider. UK consultancy Hedra is also a stakeholder in the CSC Alliance and will be active in the cluster providing change management skills, and taking a close involvement with mapping business processes. A fifth company, not an equity member of the CSC Alliance but one that has emerged as a key player in the cluster project, is Maidstone-based System C Healthcare. We met System C earlier in this book as a HISS provider. Remarkably the company has reinvented itself as a service company, providing people and teams skilled at product design and build, and experienced in NHS deployments to CSC.

The North East cluster

The first LSP contract to be awarded, this cluster stretches from Berwick upon Tweed on the border with Scotland to the Yorkshire towns and cities of Rotherham, Sheffield, Chesterfield and Wakefield. The region includes: Northumberland, Tyne

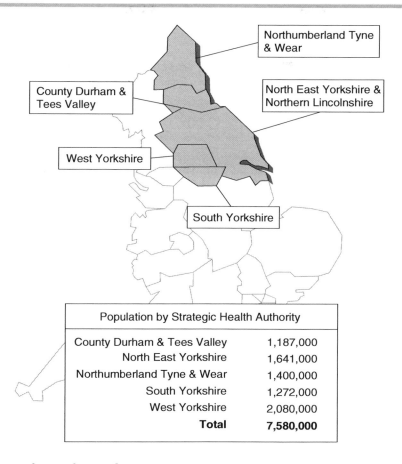

Figure 10.3 The North East cluster

and Wear, County Durham & Tees Valley, North Yorkshire, York, East Riding, Hull North and North East Lincolnshire, West Yorkshire and South Yorkshire. It includes the major cities of Newcastle, Leeds, Middlesbrough and Durham, among others. One site in the cluster with long experience of HISS and EPR is Darlington Memorial Hospital which was one of the original NHS HISS pilots back in the early 1990s.

This is the second smallest cluster (after London) and arguably the easiest for an LSP to manage. While it has a marginally larger population than London, it has fewer high profile installed IT systems to contend with. Given this, you might find it surprising to discover that, at £1.09 billion, this was the most lucrative cluster contract awarded. It works out as £147.28 per person in the cluster – compared to the £69.79 per person that the Fujitsu Alliance were awarded for the Southern cluster. The explanation for this unlikely imbalance has to do with the order in which the contracts were awarded. The North East contract went first and it set a target for the bidders for the remaining clusters who had progressively to trim their bids to ensure that they stayed competitive.

Accenture

The LSP for the North East and Yorkshire (and also for the East of England and East Midlands) is Accenture. Accenture is the world's leading provider of management and technology consulting services and solutions. Worldwide they employ more than 100 000 people and in 2004 they saw a turnover of $13.67 billion.

Accenture's principal solutions partner is iSOFT, although they did not include iSOFT in their first bid. Instead they chose originally to bid with their partners Siemens, favouring their 'Soarian' product from the USA. In the second round of bidding Accenture changed tack. Soarian was dropped and iSOFT was introduced. They join the other main partners in the Accenture consortium – US-based technology integrator Avenade, and the ubiquitous Microsoft.

The East of England and East Midlands cluster

The East of England and East Midlands cluster takes in five strategic health authorities from the border with North London to the borders of Yorkshire. It includes Addenbrookes Hospital (the prestigious Cambridge University Teaching

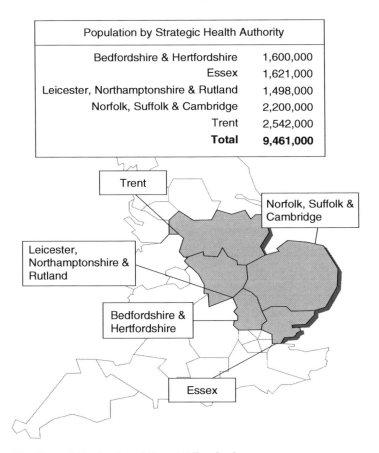

Population by Strategic Health Authority	
Bedfordshire & Hertfordshire	1,600,000
Essex	1,621,000
Leicester, Northamptonshire & Rutland	1,498,000
Norfolk, Suffolk & Cambridge	2,200,000
Trent	2,542,000
Total	**9,461,000**

Figure 10.4 The East of England and East Midlands cluster

hospital) as well as teaching hospitals in Nottingham, Leicester and Derby. If the North West is the M6 cluster, then this could be the M1/M11 cluster. It includes the Torex HISS show-site at Ipswich, a fascinating electronic prescribing pilot project at Addenbrookes based on software from French developers Stylus, and the Oracle HISS pilot at Nottingham.

This cluster was also won by Accenture (see the North East above), sealing for them a contiguous piece of geography from the borders of Scotland down to Luton and east to Great Yarmouth. One third of the population of England will be served by Accenture for their care record service.

London

When the National Programme was out for procurement, potential LSPs could bid for one or two named clusters. One unexpected result was a strange aversion to bidding for London. Calls had to be made from Richard Granger's office to encourage bidders not to simply pick the provincial clusters which were seen as easier to deliver. Why should this be? When most of the competing LSPs had head offices in the South East – many even headquartered in Central London, why should they be more comfortable with far-flung projects in Newcastle, Great Yarmouth or Penzance?

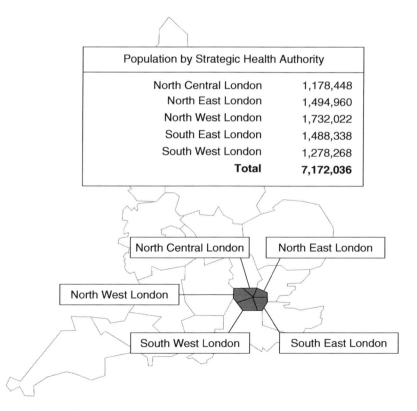

Population by Strategic Health Authority	
North Central London	1,178,448
North East London	1,494,960
North West London	1,732,022
South East London	1,488,338
South West London	1,278,268
Total	**7,172,036**

Figure 10.5 The London cluster

The answer almost certainly lies with the rich mix of famous name hospitals in the capital. We know many of them just by their nicknames: Guy's and Tommy's, Barts and King's, Mary's and George's. They make up a powerful and eclectic battery of healthcare reputations, egos and opinions. Add the Free, the London, UCLH, Central Mids, North Mids, the Homerton, the Whit, the Brompton, Chelsea and Westminster, Harefield, Whipps Cross and plenty of others – these are trailblazing institutions used to leading, uncomfortable with following, likely to be awkward. The contract for the capital seemed to have 'risk' stamped across it.

To compound the difficulty, many of the country's most pioneering HISS and EPR projects are here in the capital. US market leader Cerner, sore perhaps at missing out on the NHS-CRS contract in England, has a point to prove at Homerton and at Chase Farm. iSOFT, beaten in London by IDX, is guarding its show sites at Guy's, King's and St Thomas' hospitals. IDX themselves are in the midst of an existing project at the new UCLH hospital just down the road from Euston station. McKesson can point to the effective integration of PAS, HISS and PACS data at the Queen Elizabeth Hospital in Woolwich. Newport Pagnell-based GraphNet have a clever and effective implementation at the Brompton Hospital. The battleground is clear. The challenge for the LSP is to get the cooperation and consent of the big personalities in London to enable them to deliver the solution.

The Capital Care Alliance

The gauntlet for London was picked up by the Capital Care Alliance – a consortium headed up by BT. They may not have been the obvious contractor, and indeed the announcement of their win in London was one of the biggest surprises of the NPfIT procurements. But they put together a tenacious and very competitive bid. They are joined by Business and Technology experts Sapient, and their core software solution provider is the IDX Systems Corporation, of Burlington, Vermont.

The Southern cluster

According to AA Autoroute it is 370 miles by road from Ramsgate to Land's End. If you cared to, you could do the journey legally in 7 hours and 30 minutes. If the North West cluster is the 'M6 cluster' then this would need to be the 'M20, M25, M3, M4, M5 cluster'. It doesn't trip off the tongue does it?

In truth, the geography of the Southern cluster is not the most practical of the rather arbitrary clusters that were created for NPfIT. With seven SHAs and a population of almost 13 million people it is the largest and most unwieldy cluster. But just as the North East was the most lucrative contract because it was awarded first, so the South became the most fiercely discounted contract because it was awarded last.

The cluster includes some luminous institutions – like Oxford's John Radcliffe Hospital, and Bristol's Southmead. There are teaching hospitals at Southampton, Exeter and Portsmouth among others, and the cluster includes cities and towns from Canterbury and Ashford in the East to Truro and Penzance in the West, including Gloucester and Cheltenham in the North West of the cluster, Brighton, Poole and Plymouth on the South coast, Salisbury, Crawley, Basingstoke and dozens of others in between. The Isle of Wight is in this cluster. So are the Isles of Scilly. The Southern cluster is big.

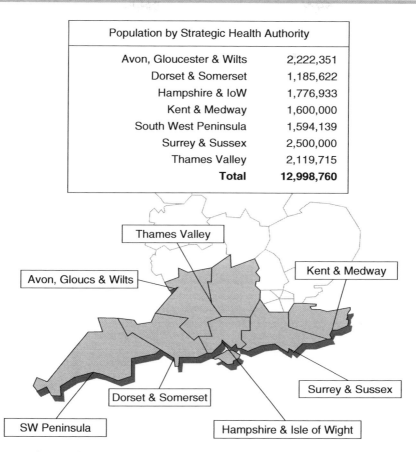

Population by Strategic Health Authority	
Avon, Gloucester & Wilts	2,222,351
Dorset & Somerset	1,185,622
Hampshire & IoW	1,776,933
Kent & Medway	1,600,000
South West Peninsula	1,594,139
Surrey & Sussex	2,500,000
Thames Valley	2,119,715
Total	**12,998,760**

Figure 10.6 The Southern cluster

The Fujitsu Alliance

Fujitsu were a latecomer into the serious bidding for NHS-CRS, and were not seen, by most observers, as a likely winner. But win they did, with a very competitive price.

The Fujitsu Alliance brings together four companies. Fujitsu themselves, as prime contractor, has responsibility for programme management. PricewaterhouseCoopers (PwC) brings technical and consultancy skills. Indian-based services company TATA Consultancy Services (TATA) are expected to bring a lot of the implementation and deployment skills using teams from their medical systems division in India. Like BT for London, the consortium chose Vermont-based IDX as its solutions partner.

Why have clusters and LSPs?

The model of five large clusters and four huge LSPs is one that is now part of the landscape, so it is easy to forget that this was not necessarily the model that most industry watchers expected to see emerging from the NPfIT process. When the author interviewed[1] the man in charge of the process, Sir John Pattison, in 2002

(Appendix 2), he suggested that the existing procurement and implementation model didn't work, and worse still, it used inordinate amounts of resource at each and every NHS Trust. He went on to suggest, 'There is an issue of capability. What we are proposing is extraordinary in scale and it is precisely the scale of the programme that requires this additional layer. It is needed to ensure not only that the technology solutions are available and accredited, but to underpin those implementations with comprehensive change management. We know that some enthusiasts will forge ahead whatever model is adopted, but it is the generality that require more support and facilitation. The traditional procurement model is not designed to do this and the scale of what we are proposing needs this extra change management facilitation layer.'

It is clear from Sir John's reply that there was a need for new skills in implementation and change management, and on a scale impossible to deliver through the existing NHS staff and software application suppliers.

A fundamental principle of the NPfIT programme is that the NHS is contracting for the delivery of a *service*. In the past, the NHS has bought a system or series of systems from a supplier. If you wanted an EPR system you would go to an EPR software supplier like Torex or Northgate and this company would show up with their own people and their own software and they would install it and make it work. This was the model. It never occurred to anyone to separate the delivery of the service from the company who wrote the software – even though hospitals in the USA had been making just such a separation for years. In the NHS the practice was for the same supplier to be charged with the implementation, and contracted to develop the system in line with the changing needs of the NHS.

Once you have bought a single system from a single supplier, however, there is a catch. You are dependent on their developmental roadmap being in synch with your changing needs. And remember that single suppliers have other customers with their changing needs, so the development roadmap ends up being a consensus, a compromise, with specific local changes having to be funded as (often costly) new work. In addition to these problems, in the past there was a dependence on US suppliers due to a lack availability of large integrated clinical systems in the UK. The changing needs of the (relatively) small UK NHS market to these US suppliers resulted in them assigning any UK NHS developments as low priority. This resulted in the NHS users having to squeeze their NHS practice into an existing American solution or wait and wait for development.

This has all changed in the NPfIT model. With NPfIT the NHS determines what it wants and the LSP decides best how it can deliver the service to support that need. It achieves this by assembling a portfolio of application providers and integration specialists, together with change management and implementation teams and data migration experts. The LSP may well change its application software developer at any time (contracts permitting) in order to deliver a cost-effective and reliable solution set to the ever-changing NHS. This would not normally have been an option if the NHS had contracted directly with a software vendor. Time will tell if this model will deliver, but what is not in doubt is that the old model would not.

Chapter 11

NPfIT: selecting the solutions

So how were the national and local solutions selected? Well, as you might imagine, with £6 billion on offer, there was a pretty tough competition. Or was there?

The answer seems to be that between the prospective service providers themselves, the well known 'usual suspect' multinationals, the contest was fierce and bloody. Huge companies like IBM, EDS, CSC, Deloittes, Lockheed Martin, Accenture, Fujitsu, BT, Jarvis and CGE&Y squared up and did battle and the gloves were well and truly off. But behind this confrontation of heavyweights there was another, more hidden competition going on. This was the contest between the unruly pack of software solution suppliers and developers – the types of companies who had slugged it out so brutally in the HISS marketplace as we saw earlier, in their attempts to be selected by the big boys as their solution partners. It was a contest for a relatively smaller prize, just a small slice of each pie; but this contest was the one that really had the potential to influence the vision, the flavour and the technology of the solution. Yet here the race was curiously sedate, and the outcome was unexpectedly short of variety. In the end, of the five clusters on offer, iSOFT with their LORENZO product became the solution of choice in three, while IDX with their Last Word/CareCastTM suite won two. How different from the HISS procurements. Where was McKesson or Cerner or Torex or PerSe? Where was System C or Capula Elan or IMS? Where was Siemens or Epic or IBA or Meditech? Any one of these might, at the start of the process, have been cast as a potential winner. Any one might reasonably have provided a working solution – especially given the sums of money involved. Yet once the dust had settled, only iSOFT and IDX were left standing. How did that happen?

The process began, unofficially, around about November 2002. The word was out that the OJEC advertisement was coming soon, and it was around this time that potential Service Providers began to position themselves for a big procurement. They began to identify sales teams that would be able to take responsibility for a billion-pound bid. And they began to try to get their heads around a very curious problem – healthcare.

While iSOFT and IDX began to target the senior decision makers in every possible bidding organisation, looking to form strategic partnerships, other HISS and EPR developers seemed to choose a sit-and-wait strategy. They would wait to see which giant service providers were firmly in the fray, and then they would launch their campaign. They would try to pick two or three likely winners and focus their sales efforts on those few organisations. It is easy to see why, at the time, this might have seemed like an expedient approach. Why exhaust sales effort, time, and money trying to position themselves with organisations that weren't going through to the final round?

The software developer seen by most pundits as favourites at the start, the mighty Cerner Corporation, of Kansas, seemed to choose a different approach. They decided instead to try and bid as a service provider in their own right. So did the giant US developer McKesson. So did the UK market leader Torex. With hindsight it is not hard to see that companies like McKesson, Cerner or Torex did not really have the multi-billion dollar profile that the NHS was seeking to help to guarantee the projects.

No two LSPs followed quite the same pattern of activity, and some carried out more detailed evaluation reviews than others.

A typical evaluation review might have gone something like this: initial contact meetings came first, at a high level. Next, the completion of Non Disclosure Agreements. This would make sure that neither party would reveal any commercial secrets to anybody else. Then there might be initial presentations by the application partner to the LSP outlining their 'value propositions and solutions'. These would be fairly superficial, but they would emphasise the horrible complexity of healthcare. Executive level meetings would establish a working agreement, and then to prove that due diligence had been properly observed a one-day overview of the application supplier's proposition and solutions would be mounted for senior LSP representatives. Generally the LSP would show up with a cohort of deeply technical analysts – people who understand computers and speak in TLAs (Three Letter Acronyms). Special allowance would be made for these people, with dedicated technical overview presentations. And that, generally, was it. The software salesman would emerge with a Heads of Agreement document and all parties would sign. There was an option, of course, to visit a user site to see the whole thing working, but very few LSPs went quite that far.

At least 31 potential LSPs and NASPs participated in some form or fashion with this evaluation process. Many did not realistically intend to participate as full bidders, but were positioning themselves for the next round when consortia would be formed. Among the serious, heavyweight bidders for the cluster business were:

- Accenture
- BT
- Cerner
- CGE&Y
- CSC
- CTG
- Compuware
- Deloittes
- EDS
- Fujitsu
- IBM
- IT NET
- Jarvis
- Lockheed Martin
- Logica CMG
- McKesson/Capita
- Northrop Grumman

- Patni
- Perot Systems
- SAIC
- SchlumbergerSema
- Serco
- Steria
- Torex
- Wipro
- Xansa.

In January 2003 the NHS issued all LSPs with a questionnaire designed to provide information on the capacity of bidders to resource the programme, and the scope of application solutions. The sections were:

- Section A – Company Background
- Section B – Financial Information
- Section C – Capacity
- Section D – Service Offering
- Section E – Proposed Support.

The OJEC advertisement was placed in February 2003, and the issue of the first OBS Questionnaire to bidders was made in March. All LSP bidders were asked to respond to a detailed questionnaire detailing their capability and capacity. This 'Stage 2 Questionnaire' was designed to expose LSP and solution capability and experience. Here is an example question:

> Provide recent relevant examples . . . of programmes/projects in which you have been involved highlighting the availability of staff numbers/ resources across the full range of skills and abilities e.g. technical skills, programme management, change management and project implementation.

Responses to this questionnaire resulted in the publication by the Authority of a long-list of 31 LSP and NASP bidders, and as expected this was followed by a series of rationalisations and mergers of bidders into a smaller number of consortia. The contest was beginning to hot up.

On 16 May 2003 the Outline Business Specification was released, and it wasn't light reading. It was a substantial three-volume requirements document that included over 2400 numbered sections dealing with detailed application functionality.

By this stage the bidders and their main application partners were as shown in Table 11.1. Responses to the huge OBS document were returned on 30 June 2003. The next stage in the process was a curious one and it took place in July. It was the allocation to each LSP of the clusters that they would be bidding for. Each bidder was asked to identify the clusters where they would prefer to work – and any where they would prefer not to. The allocation of clusters to bidders was in the gift of the Director General of NHS IT, Richard Granger, and his team. They made the announcement of their cluster shortlists on 1 August. The gloves were now truly off, and the main game was about to begin.

Once the shortlists were announced, a realignment of partnerships occurred. The disappearance of Siemens as an LSP bidder raised questions about the

Table 11.1

LSP	Main application partner
Accenture	Siemens
BT	iSOFT
CGE&Y	iSOFT
CSC	iSOFT
Lockheed Martin	iSOFT
Jarvis	iSOFT
EDS	iSOFT
McKesson	McKesson
Torex	Torex
Siemens	Siemens
Cerner	Cerner
IBM	Cerner
SchlumbergerSema	Cerner
Fujitsu	Siemens
Wipro	Capula/Epic
Serco	IDX

readiness of their product for the programme. The Siemens system was dropped by Fujitsu, who chose instead to bid IDX in Round 2. BT dropped iSOFT for London and also bid IDX, but continued to bid with iSOFT in the North West. Accenture dropped Siemens and chose iSOFT. It was a time for serious strategic game play, and some of these realignments may have been made for strategic reasons as much as for reasons of product suitability.

While all this was going on, the NHS had contracted with a company called Computacenter for premises and infrastructure at their data centre in Hatfield. This was for the stage of the process that was called PoS – or Proof of Solution. Each LSP was required to attend and conduct 'Proof of Solution' testing in September and October. Scripts were provided that would test a wide range of technical and application capability, and to add realism a range of typical legacy systems including GP systems were provided and the LSP was expected to integrate the functionality and to demonstrate that messaging standards were met.

PoS was a very demanding challenge for all parties involved. LSPs were allowed one week to set up – and a further week to demonstrate the solution to the satisfaction of Authority witnesses. A further set of tests to establish the integration capability of the solution (the IPoS) was carried out on a subsequent week. This was also intended to demonstrate the capability of the system to integrate with the electronic booking system and with the National Spine.

It was without doubt the most testing part of the whole process. LSPs and the partners were scored. The race went on.

With so many LSPs to see and so little time, the NHS chose to carry out virtual site visits instead of travelling to sites to see systems in action. In September LSPs were asked to present the Authority with the names of six customer sites who would be prepared to participate in a half-day video-conference with the Authority. Three of the six sites would be selected by the Authority. The LSPs put up example customers, and the process rolled on.

Nine months into the process very few NHS staff had been given the opportunity to look at any of the solutions on display. Their chance came in September and October 2003. LSPs were required to present their solution to an evaluation team of around 60 people from the Authority and the cluster. This was followed by a requirement to demonstrate their proposed application solutions by showing a detailed 'walk-through' of a series of scripts provided by the Authority, and designed to cover the broad scope of ICRS. Demonstrations were attended by around 100–120 representatives from the user community within the cluster. The scripts covered four scenarios: A&E , Maternity, Mental Health and Cancer Care.

Finally the NHS was given the opportunity to see what it was like to actually use the systems on offer. LSPs were required to provide a system and PC devices to support a 'drop-in' community of around 100 users from the cluster who would test the usability of the system by going through an Authority-scripted scenario using guidance notes provided by the LSP – but with no particular coaching or help from the LSP or from the applications partner.

The scenarios were built around user profiles:

- ward nurse
- ward pharmacist
- consultant physician
- consultant surgeon
- A&E clerk
- ward clerk
- pathologist/MLSO
- therapist
- outpatients clerk.

One thing was strange about this process. Certainly it tested the ability of the LSPs to mount a complex presentation and demonstration – but still there were only three software solutions on offer. If you had been an evaluator in the East you would have seen two sets of iSOFT demonstrations, and one of Cerner. In the North West you could see two iSOFT demos, one Cerner and one IDX. In London you could choose between IDX and Cerner, in the North East between iSOFT and Cerner, and the South had a three-way choice. Eight LSPs were left in the race, but for many NHS users, the biggest IT procurement in history had firmly come down to a shortlist of three.

The contracts

It wasn't just a big procurement, it was a fast one. The process which had started in January 2003 came to a conclusion in December. In the space of a few weeks, to a frisson of excitement from the industry, the main NPfIT contracts were announced. A lot was at stake. Bidding for NPfIT had been a very expensive exercise. Even the smaller LSP bidders were running teams of about 50 people, all fully committed to the bid. More than one was bringing in highly paid consultants from the USA. The team would fly in on Monday morning on the red-eye flight from the States, and they'd be back on the Friday morning flight for their weekend at home. The scale of the exercise was something that had never been seen before in the NHS, and the pace was relentless. For many it seemed unbelievable that eight contracts, covering the whole of the NHS in England, worth over £6 billion could be advertised and let in less than a year. This wasn't the way that the NHS worked! Even small hospital PAS deals would typically take two years for the procurement process to unravel. Most HISS procurements took even longer. But NPfIT flew. It became clear very early on that the man in charge, Richard Granger, was not about to put up with any delays. The deadlines came and were met and the next deadline loomed. Many tried to argue for more time, but their calls went unheeded. There was a good reason for this. The dozen LSP bidders left in the frame were allegedly spending up to an estimated £50 000 a day just to stay in the race. The bidders for the two NASP deals must have been spending a similar sum. The NHS teams in Leeds and at Hatfield, the legal teams and the consultants were all costing big sums of money. Big corporations have a term for this; they call it 'burning money'. At the peak of NPfIT procurement the metaphor was pretty apt. Each LSP and NASP still in the race had up to 50 full-time people working on their proposals, which, together with their associated travelling and accommodation costs, quickly added up to a scary figure. It is likely that in the final months the participants in the procurement were jointly burning close to £1 million a day. It couldn't go on much longer.

The first two cluster contracts announced were London and the North East. There was some surprise, not at Accenture's win in the North East, which had been widely tipped, but the BT–IDX combination in London had been a dark horse. The announcements for the North West and East followed just before Christmas. Two more surprises. Industry watchers had considered that the IBM/Cerner combination that had lost out to BT's Capital Alliance in London was undefeatable in the North West. Apparently it wasn't. The CSC Alliance with iSOFT as their main application spoiled IBM's party. In the East, Accenture won a second cluster. This was unexpected by all apart from Accenture themselves, who had quietly predicted the double win when they selected their clusters back in

Table 11.2

NASP	Winner	Main application
e-Booking (now called 'Choose and Book')	SchlumbergerSema (now Atos Origin)	Cerner
National Data Spine	BT	CSW

Table 11.3

Cluster	Winner
London	BT with IDX
North East, Yorkshire and Humberside	Accenture with iSOFT
South East and South West	Fujitsu with IDX
East of England and East Midlands	Accenture with iSOFT
North West and West Midlands.	CSC with iSOFT

July. One cluster remained, the South, and that was let to Fujitsu with IDX after a few more weeks of negotiation. There was consolation for Cerner who partnered with BT, the winners of the Electronic Booking (now 'Choose and Book') project. BT then went on to be the biggest winners of all with the National Spine to deliver, and the New National Network (N3) in addition to their London success. It was the start of 2004. The dust from the procurement battle had hardly settled, but the deployments were set to begin.

PACS procurement

PACS was initially included in the wider LSP contract negotiations, as part of the LSPs' NHS-CRS offering. However, by the time the contracts were due to be signed, agreement had not been reached between all the LSPs and their preferred PACS suppliers and so PACS was excluded from the initial LSP contract. Separate PACS negotiations continued until the NHS got the deal it wanted.

PACS will not be totally funded by NPfIT and Trusts are expected to contribute resources to the total cost. It remains to be seen how successful this will be, and whether it will cause problems for some Trusts.

The National Spine

While much of the excitement at procurement had centred around the cluster projects, the key project that would tie the clusters together – the data spine – had a somewhat lower profile. This may be because it is a harder concept to grasp. An overview of the way that responsibilities will be divided between the National Application Service Providers (the NASPs) and the Local Services is illustrated in Figure 11.1.

While the majority of patient based applications and workflow applications will be local, and will be managed by LSPs, much of the central and national control of data will be managed by the NASP.

The Spine has a number of important functions which are described below. With specific reference to the care record, essential information will continue to be held at local level where most care is delivered, with a summary of care encounters and clinical events held on a national data repository.

The key Spine components are considered below.

Personal Demographic Services (PDS)

The PDS will be the definitive authoritative source of patient information and their administrative preferences. It will not 'push' information to other systems, and will not provide synchronisation with other person-based coding systems. It will be the sole authority for the issue of 'temporary NHS numbers' for patients where a trace cannot be found on the PDS. It will initially be maintained by capture from existing national data flows until those national systems are migrated to update the PDS directly.

The PDS will have the capability of holding the details of citizens of all the 'home countries' (i.e. we do not expect someone treated in England with a valid Scottish NHS number to be duplicated on the PDS with an English NHS number).

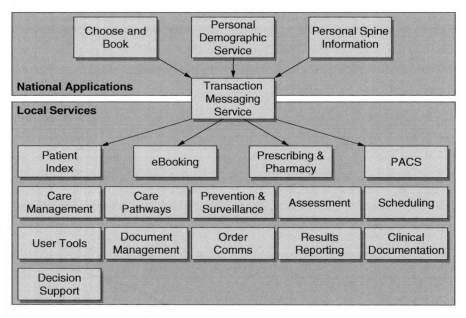

Figure 11.1 The National Spine: service components

Personal Spine Information Service

PSIS will be the home of your health record. It will contain enduring clinical information about individuals. It will be the 'master' source of every individual's medication history. It will also be the 'master' source of information on your allergies, and be the 'master' for sealed envelopes – which we will encounter later on.

The Transaction and Routing Service

This provides:

- routing
- validation
- transaction management
- intelligence
- terminology services
- access control and confidentiality – authentication and single logon
- MyHealthSpace (this will be the patient route into accessing health records – it will use 'standard NCRS messaging').

This makes the spine a critical component of the planned NHS-CRS. It is not only a repository for summary information and information about patient demographics, it is also a crucial active component of many local transactions. It manages access, i.e. nothing can be done to any patient anywhere without first routing through the spine. It could potentially be the Achilles heel of the whole programme. No matter how good or well received the local applications are, accessing these local applications in a timely manner is totally dependent on the transaction speed and accessibility of the data spine.

This is further discussed later in the book.

Chapter 12

So what have the clusters bought?

Local NHS-CRS: the eight volumes of technical response

Yes, there really were around eight volumes per bidder per cluster. Don't even start trying to calculate the man-years that each must have represented. The outcome is that each of the Local Service Providers have agreed to deliver a technical solution as outlined in great detail in the Contract.

For the LSP bidders, these were the sections that were covered in most of the contracts, covering responses to almost 3000 numbered sections:

- Requirements
- User tools
- Patient index
- Prevention, screening and surveillance
- Assessment
- Integrated Care Pathways and care planning
- Clinical documentation, noting, correspondence
- Care management
- Scheduling
- e-Booking
- Requesting and order communications
- Results reporting
- Decision support
- Prescribing and pharmacy
- Diagnostic and investigative services
- Digital imaging and PACS solution
- Document management
- Financial payments to service providers
- Maternity
- Social care
- Dental services
- Emergency\unscheduled care
- eHealth and clinical development
- Secondary analysis and reporting
- Surgical interventions
- Primary and community care
- Ambulance services
- National Service Frameworks
- Mental health
- Diabetes
- Cancer

- Coronary heart disease
- Older people
- Children's services
- Renal services
- Long-term conditions
- Programme and project management
- Testing and acceptance
- Implementation services
- Training
- Design and development
- Business change management
- New systems and services
- Operational support
- Integration and data output services
- Legacy management
- Infrastructure services
- Architecture and technical requirements
- Interfaces
- Service levels/availability and response times
- Volumetrics, scalability and extensibility
- Technology refresh
- Helpdesk
- Clinical communications
- Interfaces to/use of existing health services infrastructure (links to other national services)
- Information for secondary purposes
- Information governance
- Data quality and data quality management

Programme phases

It won't all happen at once. The huge infrastructure of systems and applications that together make up the great National Programme for IT will be delivered piecemeal, one little piece at a time. It will break down into thousands of small local projects, and these projects will roll out like an ever-expanding ripple over the seven years of the programme. In your local Strategic Health Authority you might find that one hospital is implementing a new PAS from the local LSP. Another might be deploying a new child health system. A third might be installing software for A&E. It may not look like a very integrated programme to you, and indeed it won't be. Not for a while at least. There is a good reason for this, of course. The best approach is to start with sites that have no computing at all in certain application areas, then to start replacing old systems that are coming to the ends of their natural lives, and finally, in years to come, to look at pushing aside the new, modern systems which today may be only a year or so old. This makes sense, and it is one reason why we will not really see a national system complete until 2010.

There is another level of phasing too. The programme aims to start with the easy components, and work up to the harder ones. The hardest of all (like Integrated Care Pathways) will be left until last.

If you superimpose the phasing, i.e. caused by the need to let each site go at its own pace replacing the systems that need to be replaced, on top of the plan that phases the programme by orders of complexity, then you will start to make out the shape of the real programme on the ground.

The phasing will vary from cluster to cluster, so it will not be helpful here to try to define it. It is also likely that the phases will change, and be renegotiated over time.

Broadly however, we might expect to see three phased steps.

Before Phase 1

This was a period during which the key programme principles were agreed and during which the underlying infrastructure required would be implemented.

Phase 1: during 2005

This will be a phase where LSPs will concentrate on the easier applications. Expect links from existing systems to the spine, and implementations of PAS during this phase. We might expect most LSPs to offer access to the systems via the single sign-on and unique national user ID. We might in some clusters see initial introduction of some new clinical functionality, clinical assessments and some scheduling. We will probably also see early deployment of PACS.

The initial rollout of Choose and Book will also be in Phase 1.

Phase 2: 2005–2008

During this phase, expect LSPs to become bolder. We will probably see full multidisciplinary assessments, and the introduction of order communications and results reporting. There may be some prescribing, and possible the full deployment of PACS across the cluster.

Phase 3: 2009–2010

Care planning co-ordination through Integrated Care Pathways and high level decision support will be features of level 3 applications. We should see complex electronic prescribing such as chemotherapy and intensive care, and features like the wireless information exchange between A&E units and ambulances whilst in transit. This is the stage where we should start to look for the beneficial effects through the implementation of new models of care.

You would be right if you think you've seen this approach before. Remember the EPR model? At the time of the EPR, Dr Bill Dodd, then the EPR Programme Director, suggested that to eat an elephant, you have to eat it a little piece at a time. The EPR 6 level model phased the implementation of the complex integrated clinical systems. And so with the complex clinical IT which will be implemented during the life of the National Programme for IT. Pragmatic phasing is the most sensible way forward.

Unlike the EPR model, though, this programme is putting in place this complex functionality across all sectors of healthcare and across a wide geographical area.

Testing and the model community

No software ought to find its way onto an NHS site before some pretty comprehensive testing has taken place to ensure that it works, and that it works properly. Remember, these systems are mission-critical. Their failure can kill people! A tough programme of tests – along the lines shown in the diagram below – will apply to the systems as they roll off the production lines of iSOFT, IDX, and the other software partners of the programme.

The cluster-provided Model Community will then be used by representative end-users including clinicians, administration and managerial staff to review the new functionality. Trainers and local 'champions' can use the Model Community to gain hands-on experience of the system before it becomes operational.

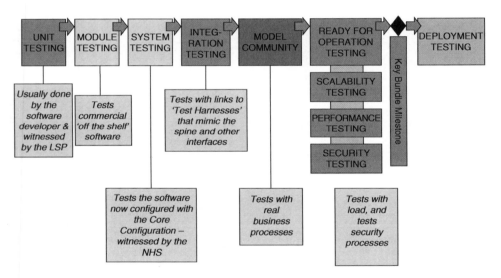

Figure 12.1

Chapter 13

The software

Whilst NPfIT should not be considered simply a computer project, at its heart lies some of the most complex and sophisticated software programmes ever written. Healthcare, as we have discovered, does not lend itself easily to computerisation. Your health record is not a simple ledger with additions and subtractions. The systems delivered have to support tough processes. They have to handle complex data types – not just numbers, but long text descriptions, high resolution images, quick sketches, opinions, changes of mind. More than most other systems, the software for the NHS has to be secure. That means that only the people who need to see your record should be able to access it. But you don't want the system so secure that a doctor in a hospital far from your home can't look at your record when you are brought unconscious into Accident and Emergency. The system needs to be usable – because it will be accessed by tens of thousands of users, and not everyone will be trained how to use it. Some staff may be new to the NHS. They may have a poor grasp of English. They will still need to use the computer if they want to practise medicine in the NHS. Most important of all, the software needs to be robust and reliable because this is an industry where mistakes can cost lives. An error in the software at your bank might miscalculate the balance in your current account. If the miscalculation is not in your favour, you might reasonably be upset. But an error in the NHS computer could allow a treatment to be given to the wrong patient. It might allow the wrong unit of blood to be transfused, or calculate the wrong dose of a drug. It might cause delays to your treatment. It might fail to alert you to a hospital appointment. It might do any number of things that would adversely affect your treatment in the NHS. Then you might be really upset.

This is what it all comes down to. Will the software do the job? Can we trust the software to work properly without errors that will impact patient care? Can we trust the software to work continuously without crashing? This too is a critical consideration. If you've ever been delayed checking in at an airport because 'the computers have gone down' you'll know the havoc that a single computer failure can cause. Now imagine if every NHS computer from Broadstairs to Land's End was to shut down. Or imagine if the National Spine was to crash, and every dependent system in every hospital and every clinic was unable to access patient details. This is the nightmare that keeps the computer wizards and technicians at NPfIT awake at night. But as we have all learned as we sail into the computer age, computers are never totally, completely, 100% reliable. This is true of simple systems. It is even more true when the systems become as complex and interrelated as NPfIT will become.

A clutch of software companies lie at the heart of NPfIT. They will share the responsibility for delivering the software that will drive the NHS. Between them they employ thousands of software programmers, analysts and designers. Since the start of 2004 these teams will have been working flat out to develop the solutions that will become the National Care Record and its components. In a book like this, it is not realistic – or even possible – to look at the software solutions themselves in any great detail. They are all developing so fast, under such continuous and intensive review and testing and redesign, that a comment made today might not be true tomorrow; a component included today might be omitted tomorrow. Whole products and platforms may change. Timescales written into contracts today may be (and probably will be) renegotiated. The landscape of applications is fluid and rapidly changing, and defies easy description. In time, of course, it will settle down. The software code will be delivered and tested and accepted, and the NHS will start to use it. After that it will still change and develop, just as the familiar PC programmes we all use have developed and changed year by year. But these are early days still, and all I can do in this section is to try to give some flavour of the big software developers who will have the responsibility of delivering the solutions that will make the National Programme work, and to provide a merest outline of the products themselves, and what they will do.

iSOFT's NHS-CRS solution

When the dust settled after the big procurements for the National Programme, there were several big winners. BT, for example, found themselves with the responsibility for the New National Network, for the National Spine, and for the delivery of NHS-CRS services to the whole London cluster. Accenture found themselves the Local Service Provider for two giant clusters stretching all the way south from Berwick upon Tweed to Luton, and east to Great Yarmouth. And Manchester-based iSOFT found that they were the core software provider for three English clusters – the North East, the North West and the East.

It was an awesome victory for a company that was only five years old. iSOFT was born in 1998 with a management buy-out of the healthcare computing business of KPMG. This was the company we met earlier in this book when we looked at the Resource Management Initiative. The young company set up in offices behind Manchester's Palace Theatre, in Whitworth Street. Their sights were set on the NHS Patient Administration System market with a product – then called PiMS. PiMS brought a modern Windows™ look and feel to what had traditionally been a monochrome character-based application, and it soon found takers in the NHS. This was a company with ambitions. In 2000 they acquired ACT Medisys, a software developer with deep roots in the NHS laboratory systems market. The following year they acquired the international software business of the US health systems developer Eclipsys. This brought new software into iSOFT for the management of clinical orders and results, prescribing, and care pathways. In the same year they completed the acquisition of the Australian Healthcare computing business of Computer Sciences Corporation. With this new critical mass, and with a growing number of users worldwide, iSOFT carried on growing by acquiring companies. They also made the decision to move a large proportion of their software development offshore to Chennai in India where a lower cost base would enable them to produce software faster and cheaper. In 2002 they bought the healthcare business of Hemel Hempstead-based Northgate Information Solutions, giving the company a commanding market share of the PAS market in Scotland. In 2004 they merged with the company seen by industry insiders as their biggest indigenous competitor – Torex. In the space of half a decade iSOFT had become the largest supplier of clinical and administrative systems to the NHS.

iSOFT solutions will almost certainly become the predominant software applications of NPfIT in the three clusters where they hold sway. The applications will develop and evolve, but it seems likely that there will be three initial key components. These are i.Patient Manager (often called iPM, the former PiMS product), i.Clinical Manager (formerly the Eclipsys product 'Sunrise Clinical Manager') and a new, exciting application – *LORENZO*.

i.Patient Manager will manage core administrative processes in acute hospitals, mental health trusts and community hospitals. It will track the location of paper notes, it will help to schedule clinics, it will monitor the location of patients and it will manage waiting lists. These are the sort of tasks that are already managed by existing PAS systems in nearly every hospital, so hospitals that swap out their old PAS computers for iPM may not see too many changes.

i.Clinical Manager will be the application behind the core clinical processes. It will hold a huge catalogue of laboratory tests, radiology examinations, drugs and referrals that a doctor or a nurse might order. It will manage the transmission of these orders to laboratory and radiology systems in the hospitals, and will hold the results that come back.

LORENZO^{TM} is the new iSOFT application that will eventually define the company's presence in the NHS. In its earliest versions it may be little more than a portal allowing all users a common point of log-on, allowing patient searches to be made, and directing users to points in the iPM and iCM applications. But in time LORENZO will be the user interface and the software engine that all users in the three clusters will use. LORENZO was designed to operate on the Microsoft Tablet PC^{TM}. This means it has had to be designed to allow operation without a keyboard so that doctors and care professionals can use it on the move. The application will remain linked to the main computer by a wireless link that will extend throughout the hospital. LORENZO caused great excitement when it was launched, with its clear intuitive features and easy navigation. At the time of writing this book, it is a new and relatively untested application. A lot rests upon it, and the pressure is now very much upon iSOFT to show that they really do have a product that can change the NHS.

IDX's NHS-CRS solution

If iSOFT was a mere youngster, at five years old when they won the NPfIT contracts, their main competitor IDX was truly venerable. Tracing its roots back to 1969, the company celebrated its 35th birthday in June 2004, a ripe old age for a software company. The company was founded as Burlington Data Processing by Richard E Tarrant and Robert Hoehl in Burlington, Vermont a month before man first walked on the moon. In 1971 BDP began to specialise in healthcare applications, and in 1978 a merger was announced with Interpretive Data Systems, a medical software house from Boston, MA.

The company grew steadily over the next few years, opening offices in Dallas, San Francisco and Chicago, and by 1985 they had over 200 employees. This was the year they launched what they claimed to be one of the first integrated

Electronic Medical Records (EMR) applications. In 1986 the company changed its name to IDX Corporation.

It was a time of rapid growth for developers of healthcare software. By 1991 IDX had over 780 employees, and by 1994 they were up to 1000.

1997 was a turning point. In this year IDX reported revenues of $251.4 million, and they merged with PHAMIS Inc. of Seattle. PHAMIS themselves had experience of trying to sell HISS systems into the NHS. Their PHAMIS Last Word® solution had been launched with great fanfare at a healthcare IT convention in Harrogate a year earlier by an unlikely UK partner – the Post Office – but a breakthrough into the UK market was still eluding them. IDX opened a UK office in 1999 and began to make serious plans for breaking into the NHS market. It wasn't going to prove easy, but by the new millennium IDX was a confident organisation with a powerful product portfolio in health. One successful NHS user became their showcase site for Last Word. This was Chelsea and Westminster, and it can have done IDX little harm to have such an influential community of users so close to the London homes of so many MPs.

Despite their pedigree, however, few industry watchers expected IDX to succeed so emphatically in the National Programme for IT. One NHS site was thought by many to be too few to make a convincing case. But in 2003, as the NPfIT procurements were well underway, a decision was made in a multi-million pound HISS/EPR procurement that had been running for over two years. IDX were selected by University College London Hospitals to provide the software for their new Trust-wide information system. The system would be implemented in time for the opening of the high profile new hospital being built on Euston Road. This endorsement for IDX in a keenly fought procurement right in the heart of London was pivotal. It gave IDX considerable credibility, especially in London, as the prospective LSPs began to look around for solution partners, and this was not an opportunity that the Vermont company would miss. When the LSP contracts were announced at the end of 2003 and early in 2004, IDX were the solution provider of choice to BT's Capital Alliance in London, and to the Fujitsu Alliance in the south. More than 20 million people living in the south of England would have their care records collected and managed by software from IDX.

The LastWord system has become the Carecast™ enterprise clinical system. This will form the basis for the software provided in the two southern clusters. The company claims that Carecast™ is designed to streamline the flow of clinical information, to improve the accuracy of information, to reduce medical errors and to achieve greater efficiencies in healthcare enterprise operations. Imagecast™ provides distributed access to clinical findings and images. Carecast Orders offers clinicians and pharmacists the ability to enter, verify and dispense medication orders, resulting in coordinated, more efficient patient care.

To date, IDX is keen to point out that the Carecast system supports patient care at more than 900 hospitals and clinics. One of the features that they like to promote is that the application runs exclusively on HP NonStop™ servers. These are guaranteed to provide 99.9% uptime, a very valuable feature for users concerned about system reliability.

Cerner's Choose and Book solution

With a turnover in 2003 of over $800 million, Cerner Corporation dwarfed both IDX and iSOFT, but despite a long and successful history in healthcare computing, and despite a strong portfolio of solutions, Cerner were not successful in winning a role in one of the Local Service Provider contracts. Their disappointment was highlighted by the fact that the company even issued a statement from the Chairman and Chief Executive Officer Neal Patterson, expressing their disappointment. The company will, however, work with BT to deliver the critical Choose and Book programme. Under the contract, SchlumbergerSema (now Atos Origin) will be responsible for programme management, development, implementation, operation and support of the service. The company will also be providing the consulting and systems integration services to implement the Cerner Millennium™-based electronic bookings applications software solution.

GP systems

What will be the future for GP systems? At the time of writing, the answer to this question seems unsure. The first contracts were not specific about the approach for GPs, although there was a clear intention that LSPs would be required, at some stage, to deliver functionality to the GP community. In practice the approach is still being resolved in most clusters.

The issue gained prominence in 2004 when GP users of one of the most popular primary care systems, EMIS, began to raise questions publicly about the future of their systems. Professor Aidan Halligan, jointly responsible for the National Programme for IT until his departure in September 2004, defended the NPfIT approach. 'Of course we recognise that many GPs feel closely attached to the system they work with,' he said in an interview with *Pulse*, 'we only want GPs to change systems when the choice offers greater functionality and better service availability than those they already use. These alternatives could include EMIS if the company decides to sign up with one or more of the local service providers. . . . As long as a system is compliant with national systems and standards, be it from EMIS or any other company, there is no reason why it should be replaced in the near term.'*

It will not be an easy problem to resolve, for several reasons. There is, for example, the problem of scale. Each cluster may have between 1200 and 2400 practices, and around 8000 GPs. Each GP practice or clinic probably already has their own existing system. Just migrating data from all those systems onto a new cluster-wide system will take thousands of man-days. Then there is the problem of acceptance by the GP community themselves. GPs are small businessmen and women, and they are known for their independent views. The early sounds of discontent from the EMIS users might turn out to be a gentle pre-shock compared to the earthquakes of resistance to come, particularly if the GPs do not find the new system to their liking.

Several options face the LSPs. They could choose to offer to integrate existing systems to the national data spine, although the prospect of interfacing thousands of separate systems may not be a palatable one. They could choose, as an

* 'I'm not a heavy IT user but . . .'. *Pulse-i.* 25 October 2004.

alternative, to offer a choice of, say, three or four GP systems that might include products already installed in the cluster. They could then implement these as large cluster-wide networks, reducing the problem that would come from trying to interface thousands of independent systems. Effectively, under this option, a GP who was a user of, for example, a Torex Synergy system would be given the option to migrate onto a cluster-wide Torex Synergy system. The GP practice would benefit from not having to manage its own system but would lose the independence of owning and operating its own computer, but it would not see a huge change in the user interface, and it would gain from the new features that would come with the links to the NHS-CRS.

A third option of course, and one that is equally open to the LSPs to pursue, is to replace all the GP systems on the patch with a wholly new system that would be operated from a remote data centre, and that would serve all GP practices and hospitals equally. If there were no risk of a GP rebellion, then this would seem to be the most strategic approach. It would give the LSP a single system to maintain and develop and operate instead of three systems, or even a thousand systems. It would provide a common user experience all across the cluster. But would it work?

One factor that comes into consideration here is that GP systems are not simply clinical data entry applications. Usually they also manage many of the functions of a busy practice, like ordering supplies and managing appointments. There is perhaps a case to be made for separating the clinical side of the system from the practice management side. It is possible to envisage a time when each practice still keeps its own system for practice management – but has an icon on the desktop that will launch the cluster NHS-CRS system for looking at a patient record, for Choose and Book, or for entering details of an encounter. That cluster NHS-CRS system would be the same one being used by all the cluster's hospitals and GP practices. But would that be possible?

NHS-CRS components

The National Care Records Service comprises a national component (the data spine) and the local components delivered by the Local Service Providers. The local NHS-CRS consists of the active clinical support systems with clinical decision support tools which produce an electronic record.

Remember Viewing, Doing and Chewing – the three components of any computer system that we explored earlier? *If* the purpose of the local NCRS was simply to produce an electronic record for viewing then this would not cause a problem. Each organisation could have been made to output the components of the electronic record in a standardised way. *If* the purpose of the local NCRS was to collect clinical data for secondary analysis, for 'chewing', then these myriad solutions would equally not cause great problems as the analysis data outputted from these solutions could simply be standardised. However, it was agreed that local NHS-CRS was about supporting the delivery of clinical care, the 'doing', and the delivery of clinical care has been refocussed, putting the patient at the centre and not organising the delivery of healthcare around the organisations or health-carers. The 'Doing' piece is difficult to do. It would be almost impossible to deliver electronically if all the contributors to that care were in different organisations, and all using different systems. This explains why the Local Service Providers in each of the clusters will have to deliver local clinical support systems which will act in a common way between all the organisations in the cluster. Collectively these applications are described as the local NHS-CRS.

But what are the components of the NHS-CRS? This section of the book will describe some of them.

Patient administration

We have come across PAS already. It is a key 'doing' system. The PAS component of NHS-CRS will not differ substantially, in the service it delivers, from the PAS systems that are already out there. The difference will come from the way that the LSP is able to provide this service. Instead of operating 50 or more PAS systems across a cluster, they will instead operate, say six (one per SHA) – or even one if the computer hardware can deliver satisfactory performance on such a huge machine. PAS will continue to do the things it already does so well – managing waiting lists and inpatient stays and document movements and all the myriad administration details that clutter up every patient's episode of care.

Order communications and results reporting

In most hospitals and GP practices, the current method of requesting a laboratory test and receiving the result is entirely a paper-based operation. Each laboratory has its own paper request form, which is completed by a busy doctor and sent with a porter, along with the appropriate specimen, to the lab for analysis. In the lab, the information from the paper request card is keyed into the laboratory system, the specimen is analysed, the results are printed out, and the print-out is sent back to the ward.

Using computers to undertake these processes not only frees up the time of junior doctors and laboratory staff, but also allows decision support tools to make the use of these resources more effective.[1,2] The Order Communications element of the NHS-CRS allows a doctor or nurse to electronically request appropriate investigations from laboratories or radiology. The use of decision support tools can offer advice for which tests are appropriate for the clinical condition and can warn the requestor when requests have been duplicated. And the resulting reports are electronically sent from the laboratories to the patient's electronic record, making them available to all with the correct rights of access.

The same process can be undertaken in the primary care environment,[3] improving communications between primary and secondary carers. Incorporating electronic ordering into the Integrated Care Pathways will be an essential component of the drive to standardise routine ordering and is an additional tool in the drive to have technology improve clinical effectiveness.

One of the key lessons learned from HISS and EPR sites[4] was that implementing the results reporting component, the 'viewing', sending the results back electronically without the more complex ordering component, is not recommended as the clinicians are getting the benefit *before* they have to invest effort in the electronic ordering – the 'doing'. It may seem a small point, but there are two sets of benefits here. There is a benefit to the doctors from having early access to results, but there is also an organisational benefit to the hospital of making doctors place the orders electronically first. You could argue that simply giving the doctors their benefit without asking them to contribute to the organisational benefit, means that they will resent the additional effort demanded of them when they are eventually expected to place orders. This conclusion does not appear to have been appreciated by all, as the early stages of NHS-CRS has, in some cases, taken the results reporting approach. It remains to be seen if this will work.

Electronic prescribing

The management of medicines is complex. It is a process which relies on interaction and integration of multiple professions, individuals, and public and commercial organisations. This complexity has the potential to result in errors during the prescribing and administration processes, some preventable, others not. Not all remedies to the problem are IT-oriented; but a considerable body of evidence suggests that supporting this complex process with technology can significantly reduce these errors.[5]

In 1999, the American Institute of Medicine report[6] *To Err is Human* reported that medication errors account for 7000 deaths a year in America and that adverse drug reactions could be responsible for more than 100 000 deaths nationwide each year. At this level, medication errors may be as much as the fourth leading cause of death in the USA. The report goes on to suggest that more than 50% of 1.8 billion prescriptions are used incorrectly and that drug-related problems when added to adverse drug reactions account for nearly 10% of all hospital admissions and up to 140 000 deaths annually in the United States.

Is it very different in Britain? If we were to simply apply the US data without any qualification to the population of England then it might suggest that 20 000 people were dying here, every year, from adverse drug reactions, and 28 000 people from drug-related problems as a whole. In the UK medication error has been identified[7] as a contributory factor in 5–16% of hospital admissions in the elderly age group. Farrar noted[8] the reported rate of prescribing error varies from 1.5% to 2.9%, with approximately one third identified as having potentially serious consequences in each study.

All this means that electronic prescribing and medicines administration (or EPMA as it is sometimes called) is without any doubt a huge requirement which will need to cover a complex spectrum of orders for drugs and therapies. It is anticipated to be the biggest single source of clinical and cash releasing benefits from NHS-CRS, and may herald among the biggest process changes in clinical practice.

Before we look at the clinical benefits to patients, let's just look at some of the costs. We may need to do some back-of-an-envelope calculations, but let's see how they go. According to the Audit Commission[9] the cost to the NHS of treating patients for the effects of prescription errors is £500 million a year (£2200 per bed per year). If we assume that, say, a mere 70% of errors could be stopped with efficient Trust-wide electronic prescribing, then cash savings for a 1000-bed Trust would be around £1.5 million per annum, to say nothing of the lives saved. The NHS would save around £3.5 billion over the 10-year life of NHS-CRS. An even larger sum would be saved from elimination of the estimated 40% of hospital prescription drugs that are either misprescribed, lost or never given. For our rough calculation, why don't we assume that half of this cost is saved by better IT? That would mean another £3.5 billion. Encouraging medical staff to prescribe formulary drugs (instead of expensive brand names) can lead to a substantial saving. This has been conservatively estimated as 5% of the drugs budget – so shall we guess at a saving of around £1 billion over 10 years.

Then there are some harder things to estimate for our rough calculation. Savings in workload, for example. Hospitals that have introduced electronic prescribing and medicines administration in Europe have reported up to 40% reduction in workload for ward nurses, but let's not get carried away. Even a small saving in clinical workloads can mean substantial savings, releasing clinical staff to spend more time with patients. A 10% reduction in nurse workloads would save a typical Trust about £1.5 million a year – so if we want to add this to our sum, we could see it saving the NHS in England, say, another £3 billion over the 10 years we've been looking at.

We're not done yet. Each year the NHS throws away over £90m of drugs that patients bring into hospital with them.[10–12] This is strange, but that is the way it works. Electronic prescribing will make it easier to track the drugs that you've been prescribed elsewhere in the NHS so that you might be able to carry on with the same drugs in hospital. If just half these could replace new prescription drugs then we can add £450 million to our calculation. So what does that come to so far? Well, this is only a rough calculation and open to all sorts of criticism, but I've done my best to be cautious with the numbers. It all adds up to a saving of around £10.5 billion just from introducing IT into the process of prescribing in hospitals. You can see from the way the numbers start to add up that it could be a lot more. It starts to make the costs of NPfIT look like a bargain.

Another important aspect of prescribing is underprescribing. This does not result usually in adverse events or death, but is at best wasteful. If an incorrect dose is given which is sub-therapeutic, it will not result in a positive outcome. There was not enough drug to relieve the clinical problem. This has the potential to block beds as much as patients suffering from an adverse drug event. It is wasteful of valuable hospital resources. Extrapolate any of these events into the community setting and you begin to see why electronic prescribing, or prescribing supported by technology, is a critical component of the NPfIT's programme of work. Of all the elements, this is the one with a real financial and clinical business case.

But it isn't just about saving money. It should be about saving lives. In order to minimise potential risks associated with this complex clinical process, let's now consider the various stages of the prescribing and administration process, and the associated risks, and let's try to identify methods where NHS-CRS might reduce those risks.

In a hospital inpatient setting, there are four stages in the process. They are:

- prescribing (this is where the doctor writes out the prescription)
- transcribing (this is where the nurse deciphers the prescription)
- dispensing (this is where the pharmacist selects the drugs)
- administration (this is where the nurse gives you the drug).

In the primary care setting, the GP will prescribe the drug; the pharmacist will transcribe the prescription and dispense the appropriate drug, and the patient or carer will administer.

At each of these stages there are risks where errors might be made. These include:

- incorrect patient
- incorrect drug
- incorrect dose
- incorrect rate
- incorrect concentration
- incorrect frequency
- incorrect route
- interaction between two drugs
- drug–disease state interaction
- drug allergy.

The associated risks described below are for the hospital setting although some of the implications are valid in other care settings.

Step one: prescribing

Let's look at the ways that some of these risks manifest.

Prescribing for an inpatient, is usually done at the bedside where the doctor fills out a request for medication. Imagine you are Jimmy Rawthorpe, nervous and waiting in a hospital bed, completely at the mercy of the busy clinicians working around you.

Risk: incorrect patient. Yesterday, a nurse went to the bed next to yours and called the chap there 'Jimmy Rawthorpe'. He said, 'Yes' because he was confused. What if she had given him your drugs? These things do happen and, unfortunately, not that rarely. You've read that 'positive patient identification' is a component of the NPfIT. You can't wait.

Risk: incorrect drug. A lot of drug names are similar and the doctor may well write your prescription out for the wrong drug. Who checks? Well, the pharmacist actually, but often these errors slip through the net, for example when the pharmacist is not on duty. So, after 5pm is an increased risk for you.

Risk: incorrect dose. A busy junior doctor may write the incorrect dose by accident or by ignorance. There have been several tragic cases when adult doses of drugs have been given to children. Not a problem 'cos you (as Jimmy) are not a child, but where are the checks? Technology can prevent these errors by checking the dose you have prescribed with the age of the patient or their body mass. This is where the real benefit comes from, NHS-CRS is not just an electronic record.

Risk: incorrect rate, concentration or frequency. Doctors are only human and humans make mistakes. The more you read about these potential errors the more worried you are becoming and hoping for an early discharge. Who was it that said the NHS is the sixth biggest cause of death?

Risk: incorrect route. Some drugs must be taken orally, others intramuscularly; rubbed in; infused. The route of administration is very important and errors either in writing the incorrect route or a misinterpretation of a correctly prescribed route, can have disastrous consequences. Jimmy will sleep easier if there are checks and counter-checks in place.

Risk: drug allergy. Drug-to-drug interaction. This is your problem. You reacted to the penicillin they put you on. You did have a drug allergy, although no one was aware of it at the time. You went very hot and had severe headaches with vomiting and a rash all over. It was quite frightening. If your allergy was known to you or your GP and was recorded on your electronic record, the prescriber would be alerted to this allergy during the prescribing process.

Risk: drug–disease state interaction. In some clinical circumstances, certain drugs will behave differently and in fact their use can be counterproductive. Clinical decision support tools can check the prescribed drugs with the clinical condition and alert the prescriber if there is a potential conflict.

The percentage of Total Medication Errors that occur at prescribing/transcribing is 39%. Computerised prescribing and double checking by ward pharmacists can reduce this by 50%.[13,14]

Step two: transcribing

This is usually done for inpatients at the bedside where the nurse deciphers the written prescription.

Risk: poor handwriting can result in transcription errors, including: incorrect dose; incorrect drug; incorrect rate; incorrect concentration. You've just watched your poor nurse, Britney you think, struggling to decipher that busy doc's writing. What's made it worse is that he has changed the prescription three times and scribbling out his already scruffy writing has not helped her cause.

A recent audit of medication errors in a hospital in Scotland reported that a single prescription on one drug chart had *three* different interpretations when shown to *three* different members of staff. The dose was interpreted as 10mg, 40mg and 110 mg! In this same hospital, it was reported that 21% of patients had an error in their prescription on admission or discharge on an average of 1.7 items per patient. (Ref: personal communication)

The percentage of Total Medication Errors that come during transcribing/prescribing is around 39%. Computerised prescribing, of course, removes the illegible handwriting.

Step three: dispensing

This is done in the Pharmacy department, where the drug is manufactured or selected from store, or it may be done by the nurses selecting from a stock held on the ward.

Risk: incorrect drug selected; incorrect concentration; incorrect patient. You've not been down to Pharmacy but you understand it's very busy down there and mistakes happen. They're only human too – you're told.

The percentage of Total Medication Errors that happen at dispensing is around 11%. The use of features like bar codes within Pharmacy reduces these errors by 80%[15] and if linked to dispensing robots this can reduce picking errors by 50%.[16] Single patient dispensing (patient packs), removes the need for some ward stocks.

Step four: administration

This is the point where the medicine is given to you. If you are an inpatient it will usually be at the bedside.

Risk: incorrect patient; incorrect rate; incorrect weight; incorrect drug calculation. Even if the doctor writes beautifully and the nurse can read the prescription with no problems, Britney may not be good at maths, and you understand some of these drug calculations are pretty difficult. So just before she gives you your dose, you have an anxious moment while you consider the implications for an error at this final stage of this complex process. It could kill you – which is not a pleasant thought.

This turns out to be the most risk-prone part of the process. The percentage of Total Medication Errors that occur at the point of administration is around 50%.[17]

NHS-CRS will have a number of checks and sophisticated software routines that will make the whole process of prescribing and administering drugs a great deal safer. These include clinical decision support rules which will check things like the dose against the age of the patient, and will check to see if the drug prescribed reacts with another drug that the patient is taking. It is early days for this technology in the NHS, but it may prove to be the most important piece of the whole NPfIT programme. The technology is already there and has been for many years. As Jimmy Rawthorpe, you might even think it would be unethical of the NHS not to implement this aspect of NHS-CRS at great speed.

Integrated Care Pathways

Here we come to a problem of names. Integrated Care Pathways (or ICPs) have a confusing name. But they represent a concept which is at the very heart of improving clinical effectiveness. The concept is perplexing only because there have been so many other nursing-led initiatives that predate ICPs and with which they have become confused. These include care planning, care protocols, care profiles, anticipated recovery paths and multidisciplinary care maps, to name just a few.

Integrated Care Pathways, as we shall discover, are really just a simple attempt to define and codify the best-practice course of treatment for any given medical condition. Like many of the concepts new to the NHS, ICPs evolved in the USA. Many hospitals in the USA now routinely use care pathways to ensure consistent treatment against best practice guidelines. It was a technology that was driven not so much by an altruistic desire to deliver better medicine, but by a more base motive, to protect against litigation. It is harder to sue a hospital when your care goes wrong if the hospital can prove that they treated you according to guidelines approved by a respected body, like the American College of Obstetricians and Gynaecologists, for example. ICPs in American healthcare did impact the huge level of litigation that was crippling healthcare in the early 1990s. But it had another, almost peripheral, effect. It improved clinical outcomes. Patients actually got better if they were treated better. Now there is a revolutionary concept.

To some, Integrated Care Pathways are another attempt to interfere with clinical freedom in some politically correct, multidisciplinary way. They challenge clinical judgement. These people would argue, 'if it ain't broken – don't meddle'. But maybe it is broken. There are cracks in the way we deliver care and as Trusts merge and hospitals become more intense places to work, it is timely to review the clinical processes.

What is an Integrated Care Pathway?

To a non-expert in this area it may be easier to identify what an ICP is not.

The ICP is not a care plan

There are different ways of planning and recording the delivery of clinical care. At the simplest level, care that is planned is recorded on paper as a care plan. It is used by the nursing profession as a way of supporting the delivery of care through various nursing models. One such model requires nurses to identify problems and their resolution (objectives) through setting goals and identifying appropriate interventions. The care plan is a series of interventions that will be undertaken, and progress with the interventions is recorded on the plan.

In most hospitals this care planning is done on paper and is a separate process to other clinical planning and treatments undertaken by other clinicians. Early computerisation of this planning process was nothing more than word processing. Data was still collected on paper and the computer was generally not updated in real time.

ICPs are not care profiles/protocols

In the same way that a series of nursing interventions are identified and bolted together to form a care plan, a care protocol or profile generally tends to be a register of events or interventions undertaken (in the main) by the doctors. A profile can be produced from retrospective analysis of all previous like conditions. So, for example, the treatment a patient receives can be based on the profile created from the previous 100 patients with the same condition.

While a generic protocol may be used as the basis of an individual's care protocol, it can also be amended specifically for an individual patient. So a standard operation protocol, for example, will be amended to suit an individual patient.

Multidisciplinary Care Plans or Multidisciplinary Care Protocols are similar, but with these it is typical to find nurses, doctors, and allied health professionals (like physiotherapists and occupational therapists) all using the same plan or protocol.

So how do ICPs differ from these approaches to care? The main difference between them is something called 'variance checking'. In an ICP, checking what was planned to be done with what *actually was* done is critical. That is what makes an ICP an ICP. In addition, an ICP can be implemented on two levels. On one level the ICP identifies the events or interventions required to be done and whether or not they have been done (a tickbox approach). The next 'level' of ICP actually collects data associated with the event/intervention and may include some intelligent scoring mechanisms.

In addition, an ICP can be just part of the episode of care. It might be just the inpatient element of an episode, for example, or it could be the entire episode from primary care through secondary care elements and back into community/ primary care.

Let us assume the ICP simply covers the inpatient element – and from experience this is a good place to start. The ICP can then have various phases or stages. In addition, of course, a patient can have concurrent pathways. You may be in hospital for a surgical procedure and find that a diagnosis of diabetes is made during that episode.

So consider an inpatient pathway. A care pathway's development begins with the identification of a patient or client group for whom the ICP is to be written.

Within the acute setting, a diagnostic grouping like fractured neck of femur, or myocardial infarction, or an operative procedure grouping, like an open cholecystectomy for example, is most commonly used. This approach is appropriate for an acute setting where the cohort of patients is relatively easy to define. However, in a community setting, the use of diagnostic or procedural groupings may not be the most appropriate. The selection of patient groups may then be based on a symptom (like chest pain), or a need (unable to cope at home). In the same way, in a mental health setting, the group may be those undergoing a specific treatment, like electroconvulsive therapy. The method used for selecting homogenous groups of patients depends on the clinical setting.

Once the group has been identified, a decision must be made as to the area, element or episode of care, which will be directed by the pathway. Imagine once again that you are Jimmy Rawthorpe. This time you need treatment for a suspected myocardial infarction. Your pathway could begin in primary care with the onset of chest pain or it could begin once you have been admitted into coronary care. Equally, the pathway could end on discharge from the ward or the pathway could continue into the community setting and on for cardiac rehabilitation.

It is possible to 'bolt together' several pathways to cover a total episode of care. For example, a patient admitted for cholecystectomy could have a preoperative pathway for community preparation prior to admission, an operative pathway to cover the admission to hospital and then a postoperative pathway that continues to follow-up services. This approach is very appealing if, in this particular example, the keyhole cholecystectomy has to be converted into an open cholecystectomy on the table. The postoperative care for an 'open' will be different to that for a closed cholecystectomy, yet both angles of care are covered depending on the decision taken by the surgeon in the operating theatre, if there is a pathway written for each surgical outcome.

Once the group has been identified and the parameters agreed, the expected multidisciplinary care can be identified. It is imperative that all involved in the care process are involved in planning the care that goes in the pathway. This does not only mean clinicians but also the support staff including pharmacists, pathology staff, X-ray technicians, etc.

The ICP is then used as a multidisciplinary record of patient care, and at each stage of care the clinicians decide if the care set out in the pathway is appropriate for their patient at that time. This is where the variance comes in. If care deviates from that set out on the pathway for any reason, it is recorded on the ICP as a 'variance', stating what the variance was, why it occurred, and what was the resulting action taken. Tracking the actual care given against the care that was planned or anticipated through variance tracking is what differentiates a pathway from a protocol. This can only be achieved if the care actually given is recorded on the pathway. The recording of care should not be *unnecessarily* duplicated. There is nothing more likely to turn clinicians off than expecting them to write and rewrite the same clinical information for record purposes. It is for this reason that most sites using ICPs are making the ICP the single multidisciplinary record to replace the many sheets of duplicative unidisciplinary records. If ICPs are considered to be a bolt-on to direct patient care, there will be reluctance in recording the clinical care. Appropriate recording of care that is relevant to clinicians of all disciplines for making clinical decisions and communicating with others in their team, is part of care delivery. Record keeping that is not relevant for clinicians and cumbersome and lengthy to complete, with no clinical benefit, should be avoided. ICPs offer the chance for multidisciplinary records to be relevant, useful and should improve risk management of clinical record keeping and, by analysis of variances, ensure appropriate clinical interventions planned are adhered to.

So what is this 'variance'?

If an event occurs which was not part of the planned care, an action list is presented with additional data to capture. This can be described as a 'reactive ICP' – reacting to the data which has been collected. An example of this is if a patient's temperature rises above an agreed top normal, an 'action box' of additional data items to be collected is offered to the nurse or doctor. Not only has a variance occurred, but an agreed set of actions and interventions with their additional data collection is activated. This allows a variance report to be run at the end of an episode, marking events that have occurred outside the plan, grading these variances as critical or non-critical, identifying what subsequent actions were suggested and logging the outcome of that variance.

This is the difference between ICP and Care Planning or Care Protocols and because it is computerised (as part of the NHS-CRS), what is planned to be done (i.e. lab tests or drugs to be prescribed) can be done automatically. The real value of an electronic ICP is that any deviation from what was planned is immediately brought to the attention of the clinicians.

So let us imagine Jimmy Rawthorpe's story again, but this time with the use of an electronic Integrated Care Pathway.

An important-looking group of people is heading down the ward, from bed to bed, heading your way. Led by a chap in a suit . . . carrying a handheld computer device – he's the one you saw in outpatients. Mr Bob something or other. He's standing at the end of the bed scrolling through your electronic record. 'Right Jimmy.' Reviewing, 'you are on my laparotomy pathway – see?' he says, turning the screen round for you to look at. 'You can see the tests we've done already here . . . and this is the operation and these are the drugs I expect you will receive immediately after the op. I will be operating on you this afternoon. I am just going to see what we can find down there,' gently palpating your stomach, 'and then I'll come and see you after the operation. Any questions?'

'Millions,' you think, but none spring to mind.

And later the anaesthetist comes to see you with the same handheld computer tablet. He is scrolling through that same pathway and reviewing the clinical information you gave the nurse earlier.

'Right Jimmy, I see you've no history of heart disease. You don't smoke. I will be back to give you some medicine to make you drowsy, in about an hour. OK?'

'OK,' you say. Let's get on with it.

And later that day, after the operation, a smaller gang approach your bed, but this time the suit man is wearing his green theatre garb, but still carrying the computer tablet.

He wands in your bar-coded wrist band, which brings up your record on screen.

'Right. Erhmm,' scrolling again, 'Mr Rawthorpe. I've had a look inside you and found some inflammation in there which I will control with some drugs. I will keep you in for another day and you could go home on Wednesday. Any questions?'

As you already know from the last time we visited this scenario, the 'one day' eventually turned into five, as you reacted to some of the drugs they gave you, which resulted in a nasty rash, which in turn needed some more drugs and cream. Had your allergy been known to the GP or any other member of the clinical team, it would have been recorded as an alert on your electronic record.

But there's more. It would not only have been an alert – 'Jimmy is allergic to penicillin' – it would have flagged up a warning whenever penicillin was prescribed for you. 'Warning: This patient is allergic to penicillin. Do you still want to proceed?' This is computer-aided support. The doctor or nurse can still do what they want to, if they have legitimate reason to do so. However, the more severe the potential problem, the more determined the warning. 'Are you sure you really want to prescribe this adult dose of morphine to an eight-year-old?' If the answer is yes, then: 'Please input your PIN number to acknowledge this warning'.

Recent work at Doncaster[18] has shown that potentially dangerous drug errors were prevented because of these prescribing warnings.

But let us imagine the allergy was not known prior to your episode in hospital. As there was no alert, the penicillin will have been prescribed and administered to you. The nurse would record what drug was given and when, as prescribed on the pathway. Your vital signs would also have been recorded on the pathway: pulse; temp; BP.

After a while you begin to feel unwell and hot. The nurse takes your temperature and records it on the pathway. '101 degrees,' she puts in. Immediately a variance is recorded and the nurse's attention brought to it. 'Warning: Clinical Variance.'

The variance can be sub-classified as critical or non-critical, using parameters previously agreed by your clinical team. The nurse also records the beginnings of a rash. Another clinical variance, but again not critical. The doctor is immediately informed. He shows up back at your bedside and asks you if you've ever had any problems with antibiotics before. You say no. He then amends the pathway, stops the penicillin and prescribes an alternative antibiotic and also some drugs to reduce your rash. He records on the pathway the reason for this.

A report at the end of your hospital stay will be automatically generated by the system and sent electronically to your GP. What was planned, what actually happened, what variances to the plan occurred, the type and severity of variance, what actions resulted, by whom, resolution of the problem.

It will also make up the main component of your electronic record. More importantly, it has generated an alert immediately which resulted in an immediate response. This was one of the failings of the clinical audit initiative: it was always retrospective. Every month, clinical groups got together and discussed or analysed their performance. And while this could enable changes in practice to ensure future events were improved because of retrospective analysis, it would not have helped Jimmy in real time.

ICPs make audit part of the day-to-day delivery of care and raise an alert when anything, clinical or non-clinical, happens that was not planned. In Jimmy's case, the pathway would not have prevented the allergy but would have raised the alarm when the event occurred.

Imagine the post-op check eight weeks after discharge. Your GP would access your pathway, with all the associated data, and ask you pertinent questions, as agreed with the surgical team. He would have a quick feel and record his findings and that would be it. Sorted.

Isn't that a better way?

At the time of writing, an ICP-like product has been added to the portfolio of some of the LSPs. The product is known as the Map of Medicine which is a library of pathways and knowledge bases for treating common conditions. It is *not* an ICP, i.e. it doesn't perform variance analysis, but it may be considered a pre-cursor to an ICP, a vehicle for seeking consensus between clinicians for a number of treatment pathways.

Clinical data capture

Each clinical specialty needs different types of clinical information. Yes, the bulk of the clinical commentary could be captured as part of the pathway, but there may well be a requirement for specific clinical images, drawings, physiological recordings. The NHS-CRS will have a component which will enable the user to design and use specific clinical data capture screens for data that has not been routinely collected.

But more importantly, the way in which clinical data is captured must be intuitive, easy, quick and must not detract the busy clinician from their caring duties. Again, not easy, but it can be done.

We have to move away from systems that require clinicians to have a PhD in electric engineering or computer sciences. The training needs to be minimal. How many of us, after all, have been trained to use the Internet? To buy books online through Amazon? We sit at our computers and we just do it. The same has to be true for clinical computers. They must be intuitive, common sense, easy to navigate and a range of data input tools and devices must be available.

Let's look at design first. Have you ever used the London Underground? Yes it's very busy and crowded, but you don't need map-reading skills to find your way from, say King's Cross to Kensington High Street, do you? That is because the 'user interface' is the tube map. You don't need to know how the tracks are laid out as long as where you interact with them is clear and concise.

The London Underground map was designed in 1933 by underground electrical draughtsman, Harry Beck. Beck was an electrical engineer, which explains his approach to the interface. It was based on an electrical circuit diagram. If you look at a real map of London with the tube lines superimposed you'll see that it is nothing like the way Beck represented it on the map. But it doesn't matter to you, the user, either. You interface with these complex systems through a simple map.

Now look at Amazon.com. Behind the crisp Internet web pages, there are numerous other computer systems. Some new, some old. The payment online probably links to an old large financial system sitting in some office somewhere. This is of no consequence to you, as the user experience – how you view, select, order and pay for your books – is all done through the web page interface. And this web page can be personalised for you. It will welcome you at the top of the web page; it will list your recent purchases, it will identify any bargains in areas of interest to you (based on your recent purchases).

So too with clinical IT. As we have seen, there are an awful lot of 'legacy systems' out there in the NHS and in the early phases of the NPfIT these legacy systems will be integrated. But for you, the user, you needn't concern yourself. These legacy systems are like those at Amazon, or are like the tracks in the Underground. Your interface is the screen – a screen which has been designed around you and your needs. It will welcome you when you log on, inform you of your appointments for the day (clinical lists; patients on which wards; new admissions overnight), it will show you how many e-mails you have yet to view; how many new lab results need your authorisation. It will keep you up to date with the hospital or surgery's plans for the Christmas do. Whatever. It will also inform you when any new research has been published in your specialist area or if new guidelines from your professional college have been released.

A busy doctor or nurse cannot be expected to remember how he or she finds the 'request a lab test' screen on the computer, or how to update a patient's progress on a pathway. It should be obvious and simple. It should interact with the clinician – remind them of things that need doing or which have been overlooked.

It might be useful, of course, if the NHS was to consider adopting a set of standard graphic icons for these actions. In the same way that Microsoft uses the same 'print' icon on every one of its products, so too should the NHS. Any supplier developing products to the NHS should adopt common icons so that, regardless of the supplier who has developed the system they are currently using, the clinician knows that clicking on that 'pill' icon will take them to the electronic prescribing component of the system. NPfIT is addressing these common user interface issues.

In addition to the interface design issues, there are also other tools which will make data capture easier:

- speech recognition
- handwriting recognition
- bar coding
- structured machine readable forms
- light pens
- touch screens
- interactive bedside TVs
- handheld devices
- tablet PCs
- PDAs
- intelligent drug infusion devices
- linked physiological measurement digital devices.

Let's look at each of these to see how they might be used in practice.

Speech recognition

An exciting development but perceived by many to be 'not quite there yet'. Actually, in selective environments, speech recognition is already alive and kicking. There are two ways in which speech recognition can be used in the clinical arena: either online or offline. Online speech recognition requires the user to sit in front of the PC and dictate what they would have typed. The software translates, in real time, the spoken words, allowing the user to validate or correct the translation. The dictation process can be speeded up through the use of what are called 'macros'. These are predetermined pieces of text which are routinely used. An example might be a standard report for, say, a normal chest X-ray, or normal breast lump biopsy. In fact, these two examples demonstrate two areas where speech recognition has been successfully used in the NHS: in the Radiology department to aid the reporting of X-rays, and in the pathology lab to support the reporting of histopathology studies. In both these cases, the clinicians are usually in a quiet room or office, and are static – usually sitting next to the PC or workstation.

Evidence shows considerable savings can be made from the adoption of this technology in these areas. One Trust[19] reported turnaround times for histopathology reporting was reduced from 10.2 days to 3.4 days as a result of implementing speech recognition. Another demonstrated savings of at least £20 000 per annum in their Radiology department,[20] whilst a third reported a single pathologist using this technology freed up 44 hours of secretarial time in a three-week period.[21]

Offline dictation mimics the traditional method of speaking and recording on a dictaphone. The tape is replaced with a digital storage medium and the dictation is then transmitted through the speech recognition software either back to the author of the text or to a secretarial support service. In either model, the original spoken word is compared with the translated text and alterations made or the text validated and authorised.

Sometimes the checking and validation process is undertaken by a third party, often in other towns or cities and sometimes in other countries. Some NHS radiology examinations are transcribed today by medical secretaries in India. In the same way that PACS has enabled the separation of image capture from its interpretation, offline speech recognition has enabled the separation of data capture from text/document creation.

Handwriting recognition

It has become the butt of jokes – the suggestion that doctors' handwriting is indecipherable. I know a doctor's wife who takes her birthday card from her husband to the local chemist to be deciphered. How on earth will a computer be able to read this scrawl?

Well, probably it won't, at least not in its current form. But by getting doctors to write more clearly and with the 'translation' occurring in real time, real benefits can be achieved. Many PDAs adopt 'one letter at a time' handwriting recognition. But while this may work for, say, indicating which drug you want to select, it would be inappropriate for a lengthy psychiatric discharge letter. Horses for courses. Like it or not, handwriting recognition will be a technology that will soon become an essential component of NPfIT, and there is a very simple reason for this. Medicine is not normally performed at a desk. While a GP might generally be able to sit down to fill in a set of notes at a keyboard, that little luxury won't typically apply to a doctor on a ward round. The recognition that doctors move around has led to the adoption by the software developers of a new type of user interface, one that doesn't use a keyboard. The new Microsoft Tablet PCs incorporate handwriting recognition which might even decipher the most elusive medical scrawl. If it doesn't, the doctors will have to write clearer, or learn to write in capitals. Handwriting recognition is coming, and for doctors and nurses who need to use computers on the move, it will be with them very soon.

Bar coding

Supermarkets have been using this technology for decades and yet its application in healthcare has been at best patchy.

During the Resource Management Initiative, described earlier, many new technologies were tried, bar codes among them. However, it was often a case of forcing a new technology onto an inappropriate process. One inappropriate use of bar code technology was in capturing clinical information. You know what it's like in B&Q when you get to the desk with a product that doesn't have a bar code label attached to it. The girl on the till will pull out a huge book with images of each product alongside its bar code. After many minutes thumbing though the book, with an increasing atmosphere of frustration behind you from the ever-growing queue practising synchronised sighing, she will eventually find the product and 'wand' in the bar code with the infra-red reader.

This approach was used in the Resource Management Initiative in some sites to capture clinical information: a big book with clinical terms and phrases with their bar code alongside. The nurse or doctor or coder would thumb through the book, select the word or phrase and wand in the bar code. It didn't work. It couldn't work. It was too clumsy, too protracted.

But that is not to say bar codes don't have their place. They are particularly useful in streamlining the workflow in pathology labs. When the sample is received in pathology, a work number, generated by the lab computer, is attached to the patient's samples and associated paper work. This enables the sample's process through the workflow to be automated.

Bar codes are also used very successfully in Blood Transfusion, with every bag of blood bar-coded at source (by the National Blood Transfusion Service) and these bar codes are then used throughout the workflow within the hospital Blood Transfusion Departments.

Another area with great potential is in reducing drug errors and patient misidentification. When a patient is subjected to any intervention, it is essential that someone makes sure that it is being done to the correct patient. Nearly all patients these days have wristbands which allow the carer to check their identity before undertaking any task. If the wristband is bar-coded, and the drug you are about to give the patient is also bar-coded, or the bag of blood is bar-coded, you can check a) that this is the right patient, and b) that it is the correct drug (or blood), before subjecting them to it.

The bar-coding of drugs also has workflow implications within the Pharmacy Department, enabling automation of the drug dispensing process with robots. The drug is prescribed through the electronic prescribing component of the NHS-CRS, automatically transmitted to the Pharmacy Department, where the drug pre-scribed is selected from their drug stocks by a robot, and dispensed in 'patient packs' and sent back to the ward by vacuum tube.

It may be an old technology, but in healthcare, bar codes can save lives.

Structured machine readable forms

If you play the lottery then you probably use one of these every week. A machine readable form is no different from a lotto form, except that instead of asking you to pick numbers for the Saturday draw, the form might ask you to check a baby's weight at a postnatal clinic, or check on a form in a patient's house to record that she has taken her drugs. Clinical data capture doesn't only have to be done directly onto computers and there may still be a place for paper for quite a while. In particular, structured questionnaires with 'tick box' answers are ideally suitable for automatic capture. The forms are scanned and data is collected onto the computer to be used as a component of the electronic patient record. Patients could use them themselves. Specific uses could be patient satisfaction surveys or, better still, patients completing a structured questionnaire in the waiting room prior to speaking to the doctor. The form is scanned in, and that background clinical information will be available to the doctor at the start of the consultation.

Useful, but there may be better ways of capturing this patient data online. The benefits of asking patients to completing these questionnaires online (rather than on paper) is that the questions asked are prompted by the previous answers, so the data collected is relevant and interactive.

The use of structured data capture forms is not new, and has been used for marking multiple-choice examinations for decades. Its use in the health sector though has been, at best, patchy.

Light pens

A light pen is a pen-shaped device that you use to make selections on a screen. A sensor in the pen detects where on the screen you are tapping, and the software does the rest. Again, it's horses for courses. Light pens were a feature of one of the NHS's greatest HISS success stories – Arrowe Park Hospital in Wirral. While the TDS HISS system was (by today's standards) an old-fashioned looking 40-character monochrome screen, it was used enthusiastically by the doctors and nurses. Enthusiastically? Black and White? How? Well it may have been a far cry from the whizzy colourful windows applications of today. But it was fast – very fast. And using the light pen, navigating around the screens was very simple. Did I say fast?

Good. I repeat it intentionally because unless the systems are responsive, easy to use, intuitive and fast, doctors and nurses will not use them.

Touch screens

Been to a pub recently? Order your drinks and they will summarise your round by touching a screen, (often with a greasy finger). The till presents the barman or bargirl with a total. Give them money. They give you the change. Simple. Fast.

But not only does it record what you have ordered and how you paid, the system behind it also tells the brewery what drinks are popular, in what combination. If they wanted to, they could even get the bar staff to add your age group to the data collected. It tells the landlord what times are busiest, and enables more efficient stock control and staff management to be achieved.

The reason the bar staff use this kind of technology enthusiastically is that it is simple to use, useful (it tells you how much change to give back) and it is fast. It also reduces fraud. An unscrupulous barman on an old-fashioned till could punch in the wrong amount, say £1.40 instead of £14.00. Chances are you wouldn't spot it, and neither would the landlord. You'd pay your £14 and the barman would pocket the difference. Today he has to select a gin and tonic and a Bloody Mary from a menu on the touch screen before he can tell you how much you owe. We may not worry so much about fraud in healthcare, but we worry about errors. Touch screens in a clinical setting will be welcomed as enthusiastically as they have been in the pub trade if they reduce the need for keyboard input and fit more easily with traditional ways of working. But it won't work with complex or wordy text entry. Spelling out text letter by letter is clumsy and slow.

Interactive bedside TVs

One of the objectives of the NHS Plan was to equip every hospital with bedside digital television sets by 2004.[22] This is not simply to make the patients' time in hospital more tolerable, but it also has the potential to provide data collection and record-viewing points at every bed.

It could also enable the doctor or nurse to prescribe drugs and order lab tests through the NHS-CRS accessed through the bedside TVs. An appealing concept, and one not without practical problems. These bedside units are normally funded through the patient's purchase of viewing cards. There may well be some frustration from the patient who is watching an exciting episode of Coronation Street (fully paid for by them) to have it switched off while the doctor orders some tests. A challenge but not an insurmountable one.

Handheld devices

Doctors and nurses routinely use wireless handheld PCs (known as tablets) in many hospitals in the USA, in France and other European countries. These tablets often incorporate additional functionality described above, including touch screens, light pens and handwriting recognition. Smaller Personal Digital Assistants (PDAs) are also becoming more common, especially for browsing records and guidelines, although the screen size makes undertaking more complex interactions inappropriate for this technology.

Intelligent drug infusion devices

Where drugs are 'infused' through a line into the patient, the device themselves can capture information about the infusion and present this back to the electronic record and, more importantly, raise an alarm when things are not going well.

Linked physiological measurement digital devices

In the same way as the intelligent infusion device, the digital physiological measurement devices, e.g. temperature or blood pressure, or even electro-cardiograms (ECGs) can capture important clinical information and present it to the electronic record for storage.

We have seen a number of ways in which the computer–clinician interface can be improved though various data collection tools.

Design is critical if clinicians adopt this new technology. Equally important is the use of additional tools to enable complex clinical information to be easily collected and not perceived as an additional chore. NPfIT is investing considerable resources in the clinician user interface to maximise potential uptake of the new technology.

Picture Archiving and Communications System (PACS)

In the 100 years since the discovery and use of X-rays, diagnostic radiology has been relatively unchanged. Digital imaging technologies will change that and Picture Archiving and Communication Systems will be implemented in all Trusts during the life of NPfIT.

Capturing and storing radiology images digitally will not only result in considerable savings on reagents/silver/film and storage costs of traditional film but evidence also shows potential time savings and fewer lost films.[23,24]

Additionally, the implementation of PACS and the standardisation of the images captured will enable greater communication of images and, more importantly, distance the taking of the image from its interpretation.

In the future, there is no reason why a patient has to go to a hospital to have a radiology image taken. There may be diagnostic centres based in the community.

The images then can be transmitted to the local hospital for a radiologist's opinion, through a local community network to be directed to a radiologist with expertise in that particular clinical area situated in a nearby hospital, or along the national network (N3) for opinion and reporting.

The results would then be sent back electronically to form a component of the patient's electronic record, and the images stored either locally or centrally.

The Royal College of Radiologists identified a number of factors which are currently making the radiologists' workload unbearable. Among them are extra training responsibilities, out of hours working, new government initiatives and increasing managerial commitment of radiologists. To compound the problem, there is a national shortage of radiologists and any initiative which will reduce these factors will be beneficial to the service.

However, PACS is a double-edged sword. One of the advantages of PACS is that the number of lost and/or unreported films is reduced to zero.

Good news? Well, that has the potential to increase radiologists' workload by 40%![25]

Alternative models may have to be considered, including the transmission of radiology images to other hospitals in the UK with excess capacity (sadly becoming increasingly rare) or transmitting the images to another country for diagnosis or opinion.

This aspect of the implementation will have to be considered carefully as simply implementing a PACS onto the existing system will increase workload to an unacceptable degree.

Scheduling

Scheduling is a funny word isn't it. What does it mean in the context of delivering healthcare? It means planning, arranging, booking. It is at its simplest booking an appointment for outpatient attendance or booking a CT scan. But it can be more complex than that.

Imagine Jimmy's episode. The GP has put him on a pathway – a diagnostic pathway because he doesn't know what the diagnosis is yet. It's an abdominal pain pathway and what needs to be done for Jimmy is already on the pathway. So imagine, Jimmy needs to see a consultant specialist at the hospital and the consultant needs some information to be available *before* the consultation – let's say a CT scan. It's pointless giving Jimmy an appointment for the specialist *before* the appointment for the CT scan is there? So a scheduler will look at the pathway – identify which components need to be done in what order and then trawl through the various diaries to identify the appropriate appointments with the appropriate people/departments and bring the prioritised dates back for Jimmy to accept or decline.

'Jimmy – we'll do the CT scan on the 13 October and, allowing two weeks for the report to be generated, an appointment with Bob the surgeon on the 4 November. Is that OK?'

'Can't make the 13 October 'cos I'm in Marbella,' Jimmy might say, and with a single click, the trawl is done again and an alternative date or dates found.

As with Choose and Book, this fundamental principle of patient choice is an important one in reducing waiting lists *and* making the service more patient-centric. Evidence shows the number of DNAs (Did Not Attends) are markedly reduced by giving the patients a say in the date selected.[26]

But Jimmy's case was relatively straightforward. Very complex scheduling can be achieved which simply could never be done with the old paper diaries. These are the real benefits of technology in such a complex area as healthcare.

NHS-CRS: local solutions – non-core

Document imaging

The vision of a paperless record is many years off and implementing the NHS-CRS will not result in a clinical world of no paper. It may be paper-light, but not paperless unless strategic decisions to discard with paper are made. Discarding the historical paper records is not an option due to the current rules of medical record retention. So we will be faced with a situation where there is an electronic record *and* a paper record. Which then is the definitive source of clinical information? Where will a doctor look to be guaranteed to have seen *all* the clinical information about his patient?

These are issues which will have to be addressed.

Once a decision is made to develop the electronic patient record, alternate strategies for dealing with paper can be proposed.

1 **Status quo:** The electronic record is developed and elements are printed out and stored in the paper master file for the appropriate retention periods.
2 **Hospitals: Store all non-active records off-site:** In this option, all non-active paper records are stored off-site. Whenever the patient is referred for treatment at a hospital, the paper records are requested and either scanned in and sent electronically to the hospital or the paper records are transmitted by courier to the hospital.
3 **Scan in all *active* paper records:** Either in primary care or hospitals, a decision may be taken to actively scan in all paper records from current live episodes and make these available to be viewed alongside the growing NHS-CRS.
4 **Scan in all records:** Either in primary care or hospitals, a decision may be made to scan in *all* paper records (including non-active cases) to be made available as a component of the growing NHS-CRS.

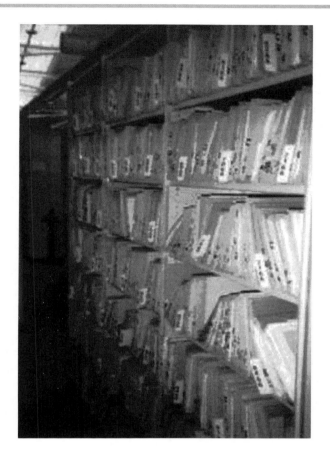

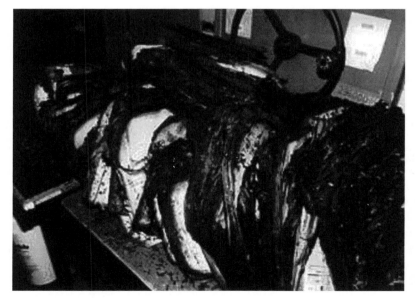

Figure 13.1 Medical records

It is envisaged that the NHS-CRS will grow over time so that all clinical information is contained within it. However, there are issues with the legacy clinical information currently stored in the paper records. In time, as NHS-CRS contains more information and produces less paper, the paper file will stabilise. Ultimately, the retention period for the paper record will pass and the legacy becomes less of an issue.

Any of the above options could be adopted by any organisation to deal with paper, although each has a cost.

Some sites may well be able to justify that cost because of their current high storage costs (e.g. inner city hospitals where storage space is at a premium), whereas a rural site would not have that pressure and justifying the cost of scanning in all paper could probably not be justified.

Document imaging is not currently a core element of NPfIT.

Telemedicine

We are used to medicine being something that is practised by a doctor in close proximity to the patient. Okay, the doctor might be behind a desk some of the time, but at least the two essential participants, the doctor and the patient are in the same room. But do they have to be? Telemedicine is the use of electronic information and communication technologies to provide and support healthcare where distance separates the participants.

Again, it is not new. In Michael Crichton's book *Five Patients*, first published in 1970, he describes the actual use of teleconferencing from an airport terminal to a cardiac specialist at Massachusetts General Hospital. The patient was interviewed via a video-conferencing link, a stethoscope was used which enabled the cardiologist to listen to her breathing and her heart beat. Even an electrocardiogram was taken and read remotely. This was groundbreaking stuff in 1970. But that was a generation ago. We now have far more superior technologies at our disposal. Once again, it seems as if changing the way we work is the really difficult part. We now carry more computing power in our laptops and Personal Digital Assistants (PDAs) than the whole of NASA had at their disposal when they landed man on the moon. Technologies we have today that can be part of a telemedicine encounter include videoconferencing, telephones, personal computers, Internet, fax, radio and television.

Quite clearly, the benefits of telemedicine are most useful in rural areas, where patients might be a long way from a specialist doctor. It is a technology that would suit the Highlands of Scotland, or rural areas of England, Wales or Northern Ireland. You won't be surprised to hear that telemedicine is big in Australia (radio doctors), where accessing hospital specialist services from remote sheep stations can be pretty problematic.

But here's another idea. Virtual visiting. This is where a patient and relative 'visit' through videoconferencing. It has been successfully trialled in the Shetland Islands in Scotland,[27] and while it isn't part of NHS-CRS (yet), it isn't hard to see how it might be used. It could even be a money-earner for the NHS if visitors were required to pay to televisit!

Or how about services where specialists are in short supply? Dermatology services, for example, can usually be delivered remotely with relatively few cases needing a face-to-face consultation. It might mean that your local hospital no longer needed to employ a full-time dermatologist. They might just contract with a teledermatology service at a dermatology centre of excellence. Or it might make it easy to cover when the dermatologist is on holiday. It might simply mean that you could 'see' the dermatologist while you were at your GP clinic without needing to make an outpatient appointment. How good would that be?

As with PACS, separating the image capture from its interpretation allows alternative models of delivery to be considered. But as we have seen, it is taking a long time to realise its potential. It is change that is difficult. Technology is ready and waiting.

Table 13.1

Technology	Example(s)
Video conferencing	Virtual multidisciplinary team meeting in cancer care Support for minor injury units Training and supervision Prison to hospital
Remote monitoring of physiological or daily living signs (real time or asynchronously)	Falls monitoring Physiological monitoring of chronic COPD at home
Virtual visiting	Remote supervision of home dialysis Nurse visits to terminally ill patients
Store and forward referrals. Sending history plus images for expert opinion	Teledermatology
Web access to own health records and guidance	'My Health Space'
Telephone and call centres	Teleconsultation Reminders for medication and appointments

Home care

We are used to the idea of being treated in hospital when we have a chronic disease. But is this always the best place to be? An increasing body of evidence suggests that many chronic conditions can be successfully treated at home by community or primary care nurses. This home care can be supplemented by use of technology which allows remote monitoring of blood pressure,[28] temperature, adherence to drug regimes, measurements of weight loss/gain, and so on (remember Hilda's story earlier in the book)?

It seems likely that more and more care will indeed be delivered in the patient's own home with equal effectiveness to a hospital stay, but at considerably less cost, and with less inconvenience to the patient.

We are being a little fanciful here. NPfIT does not include telemedicine and home care services as a core deliverable yet. But the provision of the infrastructure by NPfIT will reduce the overall investment required locally. Once NPfIT is up and running, telemedicine cannot be far away.

Improving clinical care through clinical information

Imagine you are a surgeon; a very good surgeon. In fact you are the best in your specialist area, cardiothoracic surgery; so good that everyone sends their difficult cases to you.

Flattering isn't it?

But imagine now that the NHS has decided to make available online your surgical outcomes. How many of your patients died? How many had complications? And the public will be able to compare your outcome data with any other surgeons doing the same operation.

There are two major issues here. First, your patients are the ones your colleagues thought were too difficult for them to operate on, so they referred them to you. They are difficult cases and therefore they start at a greater risk. So comparing your patients' outcomes with those of your colleagues, without making allowances for that increased risk, is misleading.

Second, you are meticulous about recording your complications. Anything untoward that happens to any of your patients is recorded electronically through clinical codes you assign to the case. Do your colleagues follow a similar meticulous approach? Or will it appear that you have more complications than your colleagues?

It all highlights the importance of capturing clinical information through clinical coding and the role of clinicians in such coding.

Now, imagine you're a hospital manager. You need to get the most from your fixed (finite) budget. You want to make sure the patients in your hospital are not lying in a bed for longer than they need to be. You need your beds to get more patients off the waiting lists. However, you don't want patients discharged from your hospital too soon or they will simply come back in with complications and that takes up more beds, which has the effect of adding more patients to the waiting lists. How can you monitor what is going on in your hospital wards? And how many new cases are being seen in outpatients? And how many of those outpatient cases will need a hospital stay, taking up some of your beds?

We have seen in the 'Infrastructure' section of this book how important clinical coding is. In this section, let us see how that information can be used retrospectively – in other words after the patient has been discharged or a clinical episode or spell completed.

How does clinical information collected during the treatment of a patient get used after that patient episode is completed? How does it help doctors and nurses and other healthcare professionals improve the effectiveness of the care they deliver? How will it help the manager manage? How will it help the Director of Public Health decide how his or her population's health is? How will it help patients decide who should treat them? How does it help GPs manage their busy practices?

Clinical information will be captured as part of the delivery of clinical care. Its use will be in real time. It will activate treatment pathways or clinical guidelines. But it will also provide clinically rich database for use retrospectively to monitor and improve service delivery.

Clinical research

How do we know what is the best way to treat a patient with, say, a heart attack? We do research. We compare the outcomes of the last thousand patients who suffered a heart attack. We look at how they presented and how they were treated. Did they survive? Did they have other complicating concurrent conditions?

Or, we may perform drug trials. We try out a new drug or drugs on a group of patients (called a cohort) and we compare the outcomes or results with a similar group who received a placebo (that is – they receive a tablet or injection where there is no 'active' drug element; some patients respond to the treatment process and not just the active constituent – the 'placebo effect').

How do you select the patents to be a member of the research trials? How do we gather together a list of patients who have had a heart attack? We need clinical coding. And clinical coding must accurately describe what clinical condition the patient has had and what interventions or treatments were undertaken.

Clinical audit

Research is a method of identifying what is best practice – what is the best way to treat a heart attack or to treat a hamstring injury? Clinical audit is a process which compares that best practice (as identified through research) with what you are currently doing.

How do you know what you are doing? Let us take the heart attack case again. Let us imagine that research identified that the best way to treat some patients with a suspected heart attack was to give aspirin under the tongue within a couple of hours of onset of severe central chest pain, and then a 'clot-lysing' drug like streptokinase within, say, six hours. (This is not actual guidance, just a fictional simulation.) If that is the standard, then clinical audit will tell you if you are achieving that standard.

If you now have to wade through 100 sets of big fat paper records to see how effective you have been in achieving this standard, how will you do that? Which case notes do you select? Assuming you can identify your last 100 patients who have had a heart attack, isn't it time-consuming flicking through them to find the information?

Once NPfIT is a reality, you will be able to search in your local electronic health records for 'heart attack' or 'myocardial infarction' and collect that group of patients together. You will then be able to identify the time it took to deliver the appropriate treatment, as all this was recorded as a by-product of the electronic prescribing module.

This secondary use of clinical information is crucial if the NHS is to deliver best effective practice. Without this rich clinical information, the service doesn't know how good it is, how effective treatments are, and whether or not they are complying with national guidance. NPfIT will deliver this capability through the Secondary Uses Service (SUS).

Performance management

How is your hospital doing? Are your patients getting better? Are they staying in hospital too long? Have you compared your patients' outcomes and treatments with other hospitals? How many are on the waiting list at this moment?

Let us look at, say, hip replacements. What might you need to know? Well, it would be useful to know at this moment, how many patients you have waiting for a hip replacement. How long have they been waiting? How many hip replacements has your hospital done this week? It would be good to know how long hip replacement patients stay in hospital? Are their operations successful? Are your outcomes better than the hospital next door? How many of your hip replacement patients have to be readmitted to hospital with complications? How much does your average hip replacement patient cost? How much theatre time is required? How many blood tests are performed? How many will require blood transfusions?

As a manager you need to know this about all your patients. You have a waiting list. Do you know what they are waiting for? The capture of clinical information at every stage of the patient's episode is essential. At present, clinical codes are assigned to patient only after their care is completed. That's no good is it? You need to know who is waiting for what and how much resource will be required to deliver that care package. Clinical information and a data warehouse with analysis tools are essential in any modern NHS and will be delivered by NPfIT through SUS.

Epidemiology

How do we know if there is an epidemic of mumps or measles or meningitis?

Is it localised in a particular area of your home town or is it randomly distributed?

Public health officials need to keep an eye on these clinical trends but such surveillance is only as good as the clinical information they have at their disposal, and this clinical information is only as good as the quality of the clinical coding.

The ability to undertake surveillance is only as good as the analysis tools available to them.

Managing a GP practice

Targets, targets, targets.

There are targets in hospitals, in Trusts, in mental health units, targets for specific clinical conditions – known as the National Service Frameworks (NSFs). In fact there are targets in all sectors of the health service.

Reduce the time patients are waiting to be seen in A&E. Reduce the number of patients on the waiting lists. We even had targets for how many hospitals should have a level 3 EPR. And targets are often linked to remuneration. In hospitals, the reward of stars is associated with additional payments. A successful hospital achieving all the targets will be awarded three-star status which attracts additional payments.

In primary care, specific targets associated with, for example, immunisation, or cervical screening, or flu jabs, attract additional payments. Monitoring success with take-up requires the busy GP to have available, at any time, information about their patients, conditions or interventions. This secondary use of information not only improves the general health and well-being of their patients, but also brings in extra money. This same information also enables the primary care clinicians to monitor how effective they are through a continuing clinical audit programme.

So how is this achieved?

Remember casemix? Resource Management? As we have already seen, the objectives of the Resource Management Initiative were thwarted by technical failure. But the objectives were sound: to collect clinical information for secondary (retrospective) analysis.

The clinical information is captured as close to the delivery of clinical care and stored in a separate database. Business intelligence/analysis tools are then used to interrogate this data and provide ad hoc queries or standard reports.

Then, managers, public health doctors, GPs and their staff, hospital clinicians, can all run specific queries on their data warehouse, or set up standard routine reports giving them regular feedback on what they've done, what they're doing and how effective or successful they've been.

NPfIT will deliver this service to GPs through the Quality Management and Analysis Service (QMAS).

Access to knowledge

OK – so you're a cardiothoracic surgeon. You qualified as a doctor, say, 20 years ago. You specialised in cardiothoracic surgery some 10 years ago. Do you know how many journals you have to read to keep up to date? Thousands a year! Not to mention *The Lancet* or other more general medical or surgical journals.

You are busy. Very, very busy. When are you expected to read these journals and circulars coming out from the Department of Health, the BMA, and the National Institute for Clinical Excellence?

You are also the Medical Director of your Trust. That has just doubled your reading material. At best you can only flick through most of the papers that cross your desk. It's an impossible task.

Our clinicians are overwhelmed. Medical information doubles almost every five years and, often, new knowledge makes established treatments obsolete. There are around 22 000 new journal articles per year, at least 30 new drugs per year, and more than 6000 combinations of drug compatibilities to consider. The number of drugs has grown 500% in just the last decade to over 17 000 trade and generic names.

Enter the Internet. Never has so much knowledge and information been readily available – to you and to your patients. Thanks to the Internet. But never has so much rubbish and pseudo-knowledge been readily available to you and your patients. Thanks to the Internet. Your patients are now coming to see you with their downloads. 'Have you considered this treatment, doctor? I saw it on t'Internet,' they may say.

But not everything on the Internet is necessarily helpful. Let me illustrate this problem. I write a regular monthly column in the *British Journal of Healthcare Computing and Information Management* (*BJHC&IM*) called 'Down at the EPR Arms' (see www.eprarms.com). This column is based around an imaginary pub in Yorkshire, the eponymous 'EPR Arms', where I meet and discuss with anyone I care to invent, issues related to computing and the NHS. Now if you were to search for 'EPR Arms' on Google or any other search engine, you would find information about this imaginary pub and the *BJHC&IM* journal. But you would also find pages of completely irrelevant information including information about a Mexican guerrilla organisation – the EPR (a bit like the IRA) and their propensity for buying illegal arms. So searching for EPR Arms is as likely to point you to arms smuggling across the Mexican/American border as to this quaint Yorkshire pub. Now do you see the problem?

Who is to say whatever you find on the Internet is of any value? Has the knowledge been validated?

The NHS-CRS intends to make available to the busy clinicians clinical knowledge about their specialist subject. But to ensure this information has been validated there needs to be a process to ensure the information is valid. It is a task for the National electronic Library for Health, which gathers together current evidence and guidelines from varied sources. The local NHS-CRS provided as part of NPfIT, will offer tailored access to these sources of knowledge to the individual clinician. It will help give you access to your surgical journals and other relevant documents.

How will it do this? Well, have you noticed your Amazon home page? It brings together relevant information for you; books you are likely to be interested in; records you may like. All based on your previous purchases and those of other people buying similar purchases. Your Amazon page is different to anyone else's. So too with your NHS-CRS home page. It will be configured to offer you the latest guidelines on your specialist subject area. New research papers will immediately be brought to your attention.

You will have to have a hand in setting it up, but can you imagine just how powerful that tool could be for you?

Technology is not just a 'management tool' – it is also quite useful for busy clinicians too!

Chapter 14

Security and confidentiality

Everyone recognised right from the start that the security of the National Care Record was going to be a very big issue. There are considerable concerns about access control and confidentiality which will have to be overcome before any electronic record can even be considered. The national (and indeed international) focus on the 'Biggest Computer Programme in the World Ever' has meant that these concerns can no longer simply be flagged as 'issues which must be addressed'. This cannot be swept under the carpet, or left for another day. Doctors have to be reassured, and a solution is essential if their fundamental concerns are not to become a major barrier to the whole success of the project. Doctors always raise this as one of their top concerns. They are right to do so.

Security

Any electronic health record requires strictly controlled access. Who is accessing the record? What is their job/role? Are they entitled to look at that patient's record? Do they need to access that part of the record? How would you feel if your neighbour, the nurse, was able to browse through your medical notes during her tea break?

And it's not just about viewing the record. Is that clinician allowed to update the record? Is that junior doctor allowed to prescribe drugs? Or to order lab tests?

And it's not just about now. Who has accessed or updated this record in the last five years?

In order to manage and control access to the national care records service, NHS-CRS, there must be a system of authentication. To resolve this, the national programme has introduced an NHS-CRS authentication process. Everyone who works for the NHS who might ever need to access the computer will be issued with a 'smart card', an identity card which they will need to use every time they log onto the computer, and every time they access sensitive information. It is a plan that should ensure that clinical information collected and viewed in the new NHS-CRS is safer than clinical information has ever been.

It is worth remembering that the current method of storing and viewing clinical information from the paper record is not particularly secure. Your neighbour, the nurse, could probably access your paper notes without being too deceitful. Trusts have attempted to manage the access to paper records through bar code tracking, and logging out of the records from the library. But once a record has been legitimately booked out, there is very little control over what element of that paper record is accessed, and who, other than the person who booked the records out, is accessing the record. That said, of course, the risk of someone sneaking a look at your paper notes is only really a local risk. Your notes couldn't be read by someone in the next county. But with an electronic record you could, potentially, access the record from anywhere on the network, from Carlisle to Folkestone. The benefits that technology brings in allowing the wider sharing of clinical information brings with it an increase in potential risk.

Fortunately it also brings a solution.

The solution being proposed by the national programme requires the use of a physical access token, in this case the smart card, and a secondary check, a staff PIN number.

So how will this new technology work?

If you work in the NHS, then the insertion of your smart card will initiate the NHS-CRS authentication dialogue. It will request you to enter a PIN number which is validated against the card by checking against the Single Sign On (SSO) database. It is just like chip and pin. In fact, it is chip and pin. The smart card releases the now signed user credentials to a central computer called the General Authentication client, and these are then verified against a national database of valid users (called the Legitimate Relationship Service) and an NHS-CRS session token is created.

However complicated this sounds, it gets worse. A user can have a number of legitimate valid roles. You could work for a number of organisations, and you may have different roles within those organisations, where each role allows you different levels of access. Remember, a clinician can only access information on patients with whom they have a legitimate role. So a nurse might only be allowed to access clinical information on the patients on her ward. But she may work on several wards. She may work for several organisations. So even if your smart card and PIN number identifies you as a valid user, you then have to select the role you occupy when you are currently accessing that record. These roles are defined in yet another database, the Role Based Access Control database – or RBAC.

The smart card and PIN number and the selected role allows you, the user, access to a specific number of applications. Once you have completed your current session, the removal of the smart card is detected and the session is terminated. It is as simple (or if you like, as complex) as that.

There are issues, of course, with speed. In a very busy Accident & Emergency Department, one current (flawed) practice is that once an A&E clinical session is started, it is never switched off and currently each user uses the same log-in. This practice won't be acceptable with NPfIT. It was always unacceptable, but was a pragmatic way of continuing to deliver an acute service in often stressed circumstances. But A&E will always be stressed. How will busy clinicians react to having to constantly log on and off and then on again? How easy will this process be? Will the user be taken back to exactly where they were on the system when they last logged off or will they have to navigate back to the same patient they were treating? The system will need to be fast, as fast at least as a cash point machine, if not faster. It is going to be tough, but security is essential, especially when you're dealing with clinical information. The first time that a newspaper hacker gets into NHS-CRS and accesses the record of a celebrity, it is going to make headline news. This is something that the NHS just can't get wrong.

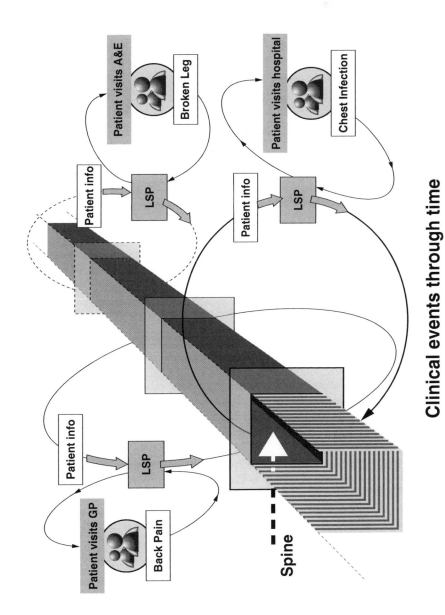

Figure 14.1 Access control by the data spine

Confidentiality

Security and confidentiality are very closely linked. Security is the process of making sure that only the right people can access your record. Confidentiality ensures that once there, they can only see what they need to see. This is a tough barrier for NPfIT, and with constantly developing data protection laws, it can only get tougher.

Throughout the NHS, individual patient information has always been collected, stored and processed primarily for one of four things. It could be for the direct delivery of care, for better administration, for clinical research and clinical audit, or for statistical or epidemiological analysis. Wherever health data are collected, stored, processed, transmitted or disposed of, the potential threat to privacy must be considered and steps taken to minimise those threats.

It isn't just information being used during a clinical episode or in the delivery of clinical care. Even subsets of information intended to be used retrospectively (for research or clinical audit) and apparently anonymous data can contain details that may allow identification of an individual. For example, a postcode (used where researchers are looking at geographic clusters of diseases) can often identify a patient even in the absence of a name or address. This is a real issue regardless of NPfIT, but is often used as a reason for not implementing clinical IT.

The general principles of safeguarding patient confidentiality are outlined in the NHS Confidentiality Code of Practice (DoH, November 2003), where it states that patients generally have the right to object to the use and disclosure of confidential information that identifies them, and need to be made aware of this right. It is your right to ask the NHS not to disclose data that is collected as part of your process of care. This doesn't happen too often, thankfully, but once NHS-CRS is in place it could be a problem. If a patient chooses to prohibit information being disclosed to other health professionals involved in providing care, it might mean that the care that can be provided is limited. It might even mean, in rare circumstances, that it won't be possible to offer certain treatment options. But still, it is the patient's right.

Patients must be informed if their decisions about disclosure have implications for the provision of care or treatment. Clinicians cannot usually treat patients safely, nor provide continuity of care, without having relevant information about a patient's condition and medical history.

How is this going to work in practice? It isn't really clear. Maybe doctors could read a patient their rights, in the same way that a policeman reads rights to an arrested suspect. 'You have the right to insist that information that identifies you is withheld from other NHS professionals. However, I must caution you that any attempt to do this could seriously compromise the care that the NHS can give you.' Could it happen? Perhaps. Where patients have been informed of both the use and disclosure of their information associated with their healthcare, and the choices that they have (and the implications of choosing to limit how information may be used or shared), then explicit consent is not usually required for information disclosures needed to provide that healthcare. We have what the data professionals call 'implied consent'. Even so, opportunities to check that patients understand what may happen and are content should be taken.

Where the purpose is not directly concerned with the healthcare of a patient, however, it would be wrong to assume consent. Additional efforts to gain consent are required or alternative approaches that do not rely on identifiable information will need to be developed.

There are situations where consent cannot be obtained for the use or disclosure of patient identifiable information, yet the public good of this use outweighs issues of privacy. Section 60 of the Health and Social Care Act 2001[1] currently provides an interim power to ensure that patient identifiable information, needed to support a range of important work such as clinical audit, record validation and research, can be used without the consent of patients.

A sample code of practice

How these general principles are adopted into local Codes of Practice can be seen in this NHS Trust's Code of Conduct for staff, replicated here as an example of the issues which must be considered at a local level:

Confidentiality principles

A patient or client has the right to expect that information given in confidence will be used only for the purpose for which it is given and will not be released to others without their permission. Without assurances about confidentiality, patients may withhold necessary information required to provide high-quality care.

If it is appropriate to share information gained in the course of your work with other health, education or social care practitioners, you must make sure that the information will be kept in strict professional confidence and be used only for the purpose for which the information was given.

When you are responsible for confidential information, you must make sure that the information is effectively protected.

A breach of confidentiality resulting from sharing of computer passwords will be the responsibility of the registered user of the compromised password.

You should not deliberately breach confidentiality other than in exceptional circumstances. If you decide that you need to disclose confidential information, you should:

- be aware that if you choose to breach confidentiality because you believe this to be in the public's best interest, you must have considered the situation carefully enough and be prepared to justify your decision
- release only as much information as is necessary

If you are in any doubt as to whether to release information, you should seek advice from your line manager in the first instance.

In practice:

- You should ask for the patient's permission before giving any information to their family or friends.

- You should be careful when answering telephone enquiries about patients. Make sure you know to whom you are speaking – if necessary, offer to telephone them back. Even the fact that a person is in hospital is confidential information.
- Paper containing any patient identification should be disposed of for shredding in green bags only.
- You should not leave a computer logged on and unattended.
- You must not divulge your computer password(s) to anyone.
- You should not look up or read information about patients unless you are involved in their care.
- You should not discuss named patients with anyone not involved in their care without good reason. Case discussion for teaching and audit is important but patient identification should be removed as much as possible.

It is important that clinical information provided in confidence is used in accordance with this code of conduct and that staff comply with associated legislation and guidance. Failure to comply with this code of conduct may result in disciplinary action being taken.

Summary

The National Programme for IT has established a programme to identify solutions for recording patients' consent for information disclosure but it should be stated that whatever the sound principles on which this is based, it is a minefield.

Take for example a patient who does not wish to have a previous mental health episode or perhaps an abortion included in any information sharing during a current, say orthopaedic, episode. Which elements of those earlier episodes should not be disclosed? All? Any lab work done during those previous episodes? Or is it any documentation which specifically refers to mental illness or abortion which are not shared?

As with data security, these issues are not insurmountable, but they are complex and require considerable consultation to achieve a pragmatic solution.

The National Programme for IT has firmly grasped this nettle and has proposed a process of 'sealed envelopes' into which patients are able to put any of their clinical information which they do not want to be shared widely. As a patient, you will be able to identify which of the people treating you should have access to the data in these sealed envelopes. In an emergency, then any clinician can view this information, without your consent. But a record would be clearly kept that the doctor in question had opened a sealed envelope that was not intended for his eyes, and retrospective approval would have to be sought.

It is in the public interest that the NHS can critically evaluate the care it provides and that using patient's clinical information in this context should be allowed with or without the patient's consent. But what about when that data is used for something that doesn't relate directly to your care? Epidemiology studies, for example, may use your clinical data as part of a study of a population or a social group. If you withhold your data then you could unwittingly affect the outcome of the study. What if a whole group of patients were to opt out of sharing their anonymous information for these purposes? Is that their right? Or is it in the public interest that their information (with the correct safeguards) is kept and made available to researchers for the public good?

And it isn't just confidentiality of patient information. Some healthcare professionals are also concerned that information about their performance would become widely available. This fear may not be misplaced. An enquiry into the performance of heart surgeons in Bristol in the 1990s[2] recommended that performance data of individual clinicians should be made available to the general public. At first glance, this might appear to be a good thing. But the doctors are concerned about the way that the data is presented. We read earlier about this data being taken out of context: simply viewing the number of deaths by operative procedure by surgeon. Unless the data is viewed alongside information about the patients under consideration, then it could be misleading. How old were they? Were they complex cases? Did they have underlying chronic conditions? And are these the sort of things that the users of the NHS are really able to decipher?

The public view on electronic health records

In a report produced by *Health Which?* in October 2003, *The Public View on Electronic Health Records*,[3] the conclusion was that the public reaction to the proposed Care Records Service was extremely positive, although people were concerned about security of the data. The perception of who would share their clinical information was understandably restricted to the professional treating them within hospitals and GP surgeries. In fact, there is an assumption that far more clinical information is currently shared today between healthcare professionals than is actually the case, especially in the communications between hospitals and general practice.

There was a tension reported by patient groups to the concept of the sealed envelopes (described above), between patient confidentiality and the NHS being able to provide care without all the accurate and relevant information. At a personal level, the patients interviewed also suggested that they would like to contribute to their own record too, and have access to view test results and drug information.

Chapter 15

Will NPfIT succeed?

Why is NPfIT different from other IT initiatives?

For those who have been involved in trying to implement IT systems over the last 20 years, the biggest difference now is the scale. Who says size doesn't matter? This one is huge.

In 2000, a Department of Health strategy paper called *Building the Information Core – Delivering the NHS Plan* identified an injection of new money specifically to deliver better ICT. An additional £214 million was made available to support modernisation of NHS information systems. This included £79 million announced in 1999 as a recurring sum and a further £53 million made recurrently available to Health Authorities from 2000. Additional sums were also made available as part of the allocations for the next three years, with an extra £113 million being provided to the NHS for IM&T investment in 2001/02, increasing to £210 million in 2002/03, with £210 million also in 2003/04.

That was what was envisaged, around £0.5 billion. By comparison with historical investments, this new cash was considerable. Unfortunately, these extra monies were not 'ring-fenced' for IT. As a result, Trusts found these monies were raided for more pressing immediate needs – such as offsetting overspends. But what is now being promised is, by any terms, enormous. It may be 60 times the bold promises of 2000. It is almost beyond our comprehension. It needs to be. We've been gallantly trying to implement hugely complex clinical IT on a shoestring, with enthusiasts. We've expected clinicians to try to implement complex clinical IT by squeezing time into their already crowded busy days.

We've also been doing it with insufficient staff. The NHS has always struggled to attract high calibre IT staff in sufficient numbers to succeed in what we have already seen are complex implementations. They have had their work cut out just keeping the administration systems going. It has been a barrier to forging ahead with clinical systems. These systems will be mission-critical. And dangerous. Clinical IT can save thousands of lives. It can also kill people too.

The ambitious NPfIT identified this as a potential weakness, and that a new layer of workers would be needed. Originally called the Prime Service Providers, and subsequently renamed the Local Service Providers (LSPs), they would be accountable for satisfying, through whatever applications they deemed appropriate, the users' requirements.

Sir John Pattison has been the civil servant most often credited with leading this new, national approach to healthcare computing. When asked in an interview for *British Journal of Healthcare Computing* whether this was just adding an additional layer of bureaucracy, Sir John replied, 'There is an issue of capability. What we are proposing is extraordinary in scale and it is precisely the scale of the

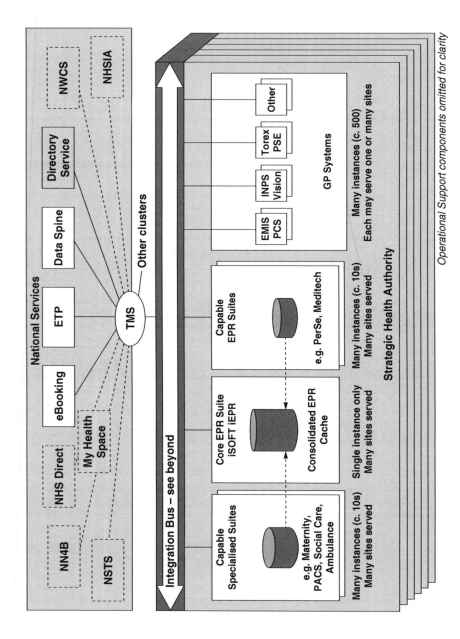

Figure 15.1 Overview of programme elements

programme that requires this additional layer. It is needed to ensure not only that the technology solutions are available and accredited, but to underpin those implementations with comprehensive change management. We know that some enthusiasts will forge ahead whatever model is adopted, but it is the generality that require more support and facilitation. The traditional procurement model is not designed to do this and the scale of what we are proposing needs this extra change management facilitation layer.'

So, in addition to top of the office commitment, there is a new layer accountable for delivering and implementing the solutions across the NHS. With this central commitment, this approach at last stands a chance of succeeding.

The resources attached to NPfIT will ensure a more robust implementation approach and not be restricted by patchy project funding. It will ensure the national IT infrastructure is embedded within the infrastructure of the NHS and as long as NPfIT continues to be mindful of why IT projects have failed in the past, then NPfIT should not fail.

Finally, there is one very fundamental way, of course, that NPfIT differs from nearly every other government computer project. When the pessimists shake their heads and warn that every government-sponsored IT project ends in failure (which is patently untrue, of course, there have been plenty that haven't), it is worth noting that in general, high profile failures have occurred when all the risk of success or failure has rested on a single system – a single successful go-live. The ill-fated system at the Child Support Agency was, after all, effectively a single key system. If the project outcome is a single system, and that system doesn't work or doesn't meet the needs of users, then the whole project fails. But NPfIT will have thousands of go-lives. Hundreds of these will be for fairly mundane PAS functionality that the NHS has done countless times before. These really ought to work. Then there will be a gradual ramping up of functionality over hundreds of sites over several years. At what point does the system qualify as a success or a failure? The only single point of failure, and the one that will attract the most attention if it fails, is the spine.

So we come to the £30 billion question. Will it work?

If NPfIT is about getting the best deal for IT infrastructure for the NHS then, yes, it will be a success. The NHS was a huge spender on IT before the national programme started. Now it gets more, it gets it delivered as a service, and it gets it all at a very keen price. It will get several hundred PAS systems, clinical systems, and all sorts of associated applications delivered down a pipe to the bedside.

So let's try a tougher question. Will all the software and applications work in the way that they are meant to work? Will the spine integrate seamlessly with systems in the five clusters? Will the security and confidentiality work to everyone's satisfaction? The answer to this question is probably 'eventually'. So long as the momentum is maintained and the funding is sustained, then one day it will all come together. There is, after all, very little in the programme that is totally conceptually new. But it may all take a lot longer than the NHS expects. New software always seems to take longer to design, build and test than anyone expects. This is an ambitious programme, and there are many obstacles in the path. The main software developers have a lot of code to write. I would expect to see slippages, renegotiations of deadlines, a general downplaying of expectations, and a long hard slog by the service providers, the software developers, and the NHS alike before it all starts to come together. There will certainly be scare stories along the way. The press will gather around every hint of failure and will predict catastrophe. But in the end, this isn't rocket science. It will work because it has to work. The day will come when the systems are in and the project will be signed off. Of course, by then there will be new challenges, new technologies, new obstacles. But that will be tomorrow's problem. Another rainbow.

But perhaps even this wasn't the question that you wanted answering. If NPfIT is about changing the way healthcare is delivered, then there is a third answer to the question 'will NPfIT succeed?' It will struggle. 'That's not what NPfIT is about,' I can hear from some readers, and true, the programme's remit isn't to change the world, just to deliver as a service to the NHS, an IT infrastructure for the NHS to use as it chooses. The programme is branded and perceived as a technology initiative. It *is* a technology initiative. Yet this perception could be its undoing. People might assume it to be non-clinical. It could become another big PAS project. And that would be a shame. The deals that have been negotiated by the national programme are there to ensure that the NHS has access to cutting-edge technology after years of 'playing around' with IT. But will clinicians see the opportunities to change the way the NHS is delivered? Will this change be an opportunity to them or a threat?

The key purpose of the NHS is to deliver effective clinical care. Technology will offer alternative ways of delivering that care so NPfIT is, whether it likes it or not, central to the modernisation of the delivery of clinical care. This is not just about having an electronic record. It is far deeper and grander than that. It is about supporting clinical care with IT, and when you support clinical care with IT, you can then use that technology to influence how that care is delivered.

Electronic records

That an electronic record would be a great asset to the delivery of clinical care is not in doubt. Clinical failures have previously been blamed on illegible handwriting (so much so that in America, some states are considering banning doctors from handwriting), on breakdown in communications between health carers and other organisations (e.g. social services) and on the treatment of patients outside of the natural community. An electronic record will bring undoubted benefits in this area.

If we want to understand how IT can change healthcare delivery, let's take, as an example, the current process of prescribing drugs on a hospital ward. The junior doctor writes the drug order on the drug chart. The nurse, on reading this order, administers the drugs appropriately. If we were simply to require an electronic record of that process, the paper drug charts could be collected every night and data input clerks could record the drugs prescribed for each patient on a computer. Alternatively, the drug charts could be scanned into a computer. In both cases you would have an *electronic record* of the drugs prescribed. However, what you will have lost is the opportunity to *influence* what was prescribed. Bates *et al.* have clearly demonstrated that computer decision support can enhance the quality of care, can reduce drug-related errors, and can cut down the number of inappropriate laboratory investigations by supporting these doctors in those clinical processes.[1,2] Checking the drugs prescribed against the drugs the patient is currently taking, checking for potential drug–drug interactions, checking the dose of the drug proposed against the patient's body mass, checking that the drug intended is one the hospital recommends within its drug formulary or that the patient does not have a sensitivity to the prescribed drugs: these are the *real* benefits of using computers – in assisting the clinical process. Not mandating it, but assisting it. And the by-product is an electronic record, not only of what has been prescribed, but of who prescribed it and whether or not the drug was administered, when, how and by whom. The record in electronic format is important, but only as a secondary process and as a by-product of the delivery of clinical care.

Long-term view

But hang on a minute, let's take a longer term view of the NHS. If we were to maintain the status quo in the health service, maintain the workflow between primary care and secondary care, continue with the age-old organisation boundaries that have served us so well for so long, there would be little need for the grand vision of a national integrated care record. It is consistently reported that more than 95% of clinical care is delivered within a relatively small clinical community. And of that care delivered locally, 90% is delivered in a primary care or community setting. We have our own GP or family doctor who treats us or refers us to a specialist in our local hospital. A model which has stood the test of time and has changed little in its 60 years. The communication of clinical information within that simple workflow works OK. Not good, but not danger-ous. So if the implementation of these expensive computers is to improve clinical effectiveness, then the national record is really only going to be noticed in 5% of cases, cases where care is *not* delivered within that well tried and trusted clinical workflow.

However, what makes the integrated record a necessity is that a new model of care has been proposed that can *not* be delivered with the traditional model. There are many drivers for this change:

- **New GP contracts:** We will not be guaranteed to see our own doctor but one from a co-operative of doctors. Sharing the paper record envelope (introduced during Lloyd George's reign as Prime Minister and therefore known colloqui-ally known as the 'Lloyd George') will not sustain this model.
- **Shifting work from doctors to nurses:** Clinical processes previously the sole domain of the doctors, are now being undertaken by nurses, and other clinicians, both in hospital and in the community.
- **Shifting the balance of power:** Delivering clinical care as close to the patient as possible will result in more preventative and interventionist care being delivered in the community or in the home, and not just by doctors.
- **Purchasing care:** The PCT's ability to purchase care from non-traditional care providers including private hospitals, specialist clinics, eye laser centres and diagnostic/treatment centres.
- **GP specialists:** Increased numbers of GP specialists reducing the need to refer patients to hospital at all.

- **Nurse specialists:** Emergence of the 'super-nurses' in the community, dealing with specific clinical conditions. A considerable number of Chronic Obstructive Pulmonary Disease (COPD) cases can be treated as effectively in the patient's own home and at a considerable reduction in cost.
- **Patient choice:** Giving the population 'choice' is an objective of the current government. Choice as to whether you are treated by your local hospital, local GP, walk-in centre or diagnostic treatment centre requires there must be a single definitive record of that care, wherever it is delivered.
- **An end to paper:** The static, paper-based record has been a significant barrier to any new ways of working. The NHS-CRS data spine will enable considerable redesign of the NHS.

There is an increasing demand for accountability of all working in the NHS. Although successive initiatives have attempted to instil a more rigorous approach to monitoring the effectiveness of care given, this has generally been undertaken locally and behind closed doors. A central, structured database of clinical information will enable third-party regulation to be achieved by organisations like the Healthcare Commission.

The national record is a prerequisite for change, but with the existing organisational model there is no business case for the investment. There is a considerable current clinical business case, however, for the implementation of systems to support the clinicians in what they do. It may have been more pragmatic to implement these local clinical systems first and in time pull their outputs together in a large single national database. NPfIT, however, have chosen to start with the data spine. In its early days of existence, 'spine' seems like an overstatement: a couple of vertebrae more like. But an area of real concern is the decision to insist that any clinical intervention (supported by the local NHS-CRS) is undertaken *through* the spine. A better model may have been to insist on a standardised output from the systems which would locally manage the transactions.

Single log-on and authentication at a national level is a real potential bottleneck at a time when we are moving to systems which will become mission-critical. If it takes an age to log on and be authenticated, then this could result in user apathy. Worse still, clinicians could try to find ways to delegate the tasks to other more junior personnel. The whole foundation of user consent to the system could start to crumble.

There are concerns that the widespread adoption of web technology in these mission-critical clinical systems could also bring delays. Web pages need to refresh and this 'hanging' could be perceived as a frustrating delay. Evidence has shown us that clinicians need sub-second rapid response rates from their clinical applications if we are to keep their support. Now all this may be doing the software application providers a disservice, after all no one expects that their final product will not be fit for purpose. But no one really knows – yet.

Another area of potential concern is how *generic* the LSPs' NHS-CRS solution is going to be. We have witnessed first-hand, or at least through this book, the success at sites such as Greenwich, Burton, Winchester and Wirral. Their success was not easily replicated in other sites, even with the same IT system. Why? Because the Burtons and Wirrals and Winchesters and Greenwichs had a very tailored solution. It was 'moulded' around their work practices, and the systems fit like a glove.

Will NPfIT be able to offer a similar local tailoring service or will it be 'one size fits all?' And how successful will that be? Will it result in a dumbing down of functionality in order to get consensus?

The final major concern is not a technology one, but a clinical one, stimulated by the implementation of technology.

During any preimplementation analysis phase of a large computer project, workflow processes are identified and compared.

Imagine the workflow involved in an Integrated Care Pathway.

Imagine all the healthcare workers who input into a single pathway.

Imagine four different surgeons who have four completely different ways of treating the same condition.

Easy, you say, just look at the evidence for which is the *correct* way to treat that condition and get them all to do it that way.

Mmmm. That is the challenge. Changing existing work practices which have evolved over many years will not be easy. Implementing the technology is relatively easy compared to getting agreement on changing clinical practice and implementing Integrated Care Pathways.

Simply imposing pathways on these guys (and gals) will not work.

So, back to our £30 billion question once again. Will NPfIT work? Yes, it will deliver the technology to the NHS. But for the NHS to grab this opportunity, the clinicians need considerable encouragement, a clearer idea of what will be delivered and evidence of benefit. Take one aspect of this huge programme of work: clinical coding. Here is a whole raft of issues. Many have yet to be identified, let alone resolved, if real-time clinical coding is to be achieved. Yet this is essential if intelligent decision support tools are to be used. Or take another aspect: security and confidentiality. This may also prove to be a show-stopper and although NPfIT have firmly grasped this nettle, the problem has not yet gone away. And what if there is a change of Government? Would this ambitious programme continue to be supported?

It all begs the question, could there have been a better way to do it? We will probably never know. Like it or not, NPfIT is now the only game in town. As I said in the opening pages of this book, this is a huge and complex undertaking. It is essential for the NHS that this technology is implemented successfully. It must not fail.

In order to reduce the risk of failure, it is worth identifying those risks and barriers and identifying a strategy for minimising or eradicating them.

What are the barriers to success?

NPfIT is the biggest IT programme in the world. Why should this computer programme be any different than those that have gone before and failed?

Let's look at why computer projects fail. In *Crash: Ten easy ways to avoid a computer disaster* by Tony Collins, 10 themes have been identified which appear to occur in all disasters (reproduced here *verbatim* with permission):[3]

1 A tendency to be overambitious.
2 A feeling among computer managers that they should know it all and can't admit it when they don't.

3 A belief among the entire project team that computerisation must be a good thing, and to suspect otherwise is an Orwellian thoughtcrime.

4 A Chief Executive who is in the best position to judge a computer project because he knows nothing about computers but fails to intervene – because he knows nothing about computers.

5 A readiness to accept 'it'll be alright on the night' assurances from suppliers – assurances that suppliers studiously avoid writing down.

6 An overreliance on consultants who, like some vets, may have a financial interest in prolonging ills.

7 An avoidance of cheap, proven, off-the-shelf packages in favour of costly, unproven, custom-built software; or worse, the tailoring of a standard proven package.

8 An unwillingness by middle and senior management to impart bad news to the board – mainly because the board will make known its resentment of anyone who tries.

9 The buck stops nowhere.

10 A mistaken belief that the contract makes it easy to sue the supplier if all goes wrong.

Collins goes on to say that, 'people become so absorbed in the technology that they lose sight or even interest in the benefits to the business'.

Look at each and every one of these 10 factors. Have they all been addressed by NPfIT?

Even if all the above sins are avoided, the result can still be a disaster. Why? Is it apathy? Disinterest? Or is it a scepticism that what is promised will never be delivered and so it's safer to keep your head down and carry on as before because, at the end of the day, doctors and nurses and others will still have to treat patients regardless of these fancy systems. Wait till it blows over, just carry on as before. What goes around comes around.

And on top of all that, there's resistance to change . . .

Resistance to change

NPfIT has addressed most of the 10 deadly sins, but resistance to change will still need to be addressed. Rick Maurer in *Beyond the Wall of Resistance* suggests that resistance is not necessarily a bad thing.[4] It is at least a force, an energy which, if redirected, can be a useful energy.

He goes on to propose three different types of resistance (repeated here with permission).

- level 1 resistance
- level 2 resistance
- level 3 resistance.

Level 1 resistance is a low-grade resistance where there is no hidden agenda. People are simply opposed to the idea for any number of reasons: lack of information, disagreement with the idea itself, lack of exposure or confusion.

Level 2 resistance is an emotional physiological reaction to change. Blood pressure rises, adrenaline flows, pulse increases. It is uncontrollable and based on fear that they may lose face, friends, even their jobs. Level 2 resistance can be triggered without conscious awareness.

Level 3 resistance is deeply entrenched and is bigger than the ideas at hand. People are not resisting the idea – in fact, they may love the idea itself – they are resisting you. They may resist because of their history with you or they may oppose what you represent.

Working with resistance

In working with resistance, it is critical that your strategy matches the type of resistance you are facing.

To deal with a level 1, people need to be given more information – newsletters, e-mails, memos, videos, etc. They need to gain an understanding of the proposed change. They must see ideas from their perspectives and must have a clear understanding about how the change impacts them. People also need a chance to engage with the information. They need a chance to chew on what they hear. They must feel that they have an opportunity to make a contribution to the idea or warn of potential pitfalls.

The tactics used for level 1 will not work with a level 2 resistance. You need to engage people in ways that address their fears. To move beyond this resistance, don't battle it – embrace it. Listen to those who resist change and try to understand how they feel and why they feel that way. Then try to find common ground, incorporating their concerns.

Overcoming level 3 resistance is the most problematic as there is a deep seated mistrust of you personally or who you represent. Overcoming this type of resistance will require continual work on relationships. Begin small. Candid conversation is important. Support yourself and be calm, get people deeply involved in changes that affect them, be prepared for setbacks, be prepared to walk away.

More detail on overcoming resistance can be found in Rick Maurer's book *Beyond the Wall of Resistance*.

It seems an almost universal truth that in any organisation there are enthusiasts, there are pragmatists, there are cynics and there are grumpy 'I'll never change as long as I've a breath in my body' folk. It has been suggested that an enthusiast will never ever convince a cynic of the value of change, or of the value of computerising a process. But a pragmatist can be convinced of its value if given evidence. And – this is the good bit – a cynic may be convinced by a pragmatist.

What about the grumpy folk, I hear you ask. Wait till they retire. Or get the cynics to convince them.

So why do computer projects fail? Many different reasons, but probably the most difficult challenge is the people issues. Resistance. And the way to overcome resistance is to engage with those who are expected to use such technology in the ways described above.

The need for clinical engagement

The NHS National Programme for IT risks failure if it does not engage the medical profession, the British Medical Association's IT committee warned in November 2004. It was one salvo in a barrage of warnings from doctors concerned that their opinions were not being sought in this huge national programme. 'The health service should learn from past government IT projects where poor user consultation has contributed to failure,' said John Powell, who chaired the BMA committee. 'The programme should support healthcare workers in delivering a better service to their patients. We hope that improvements to IT systems will reduce the administrative burden on doctors so they can spend more time treating patients,' Powell said.

Of all the potential pitfalls that might await this ambitious programme, the most serious must be the real possibility that doctors will simply refuse to use the system. When a bank introduces a new computer this just isn't a concern. Nobody worries that the bank tellers will indulge some grand rebellion and insist on using their paper ledgers. Nobody worried when the new air traffic control system went live that some airline pilots might boycott the system and navigate their way by looking out of the cockpit window. But doctors are a whole different constituency and they have a lot of very real concerns, about security and confidentiality and usability. They might decide that their concerns are not sufficiently addressed by the new computer, and they might simply not use it.

Now in a sense this is only a concern for NPfIT if the doctors are organised. This is because, for an individual doctor, the use of NHS-CRS will not be discretionary. You may want to read that last sentence again. Doctors, alone, will not be able to choose to boycott the system if they want to practise medicine. This won't be because the thought-police will hunt them down, it will be because the processes of the NHS just won't work unless they are computer users. It won't happen all at once, but it will happen. Soon, if you are a doctor, you will not be able to look at your patient's notes unless you look at the computer. OK, you say, what if the doctor decides to keep his own paper notes? Well, you won't be able to see the patient's laboratory results or X-ray reports. Worse than that, you won't be able to order the lab tests or X-rays in the first place. You won't be able to refer your patient to a consultant, or admit your patient into a ward. You won't be able to prescribe a drug. In short, you will not be able to work as a doctor in the NHS if you don't use the computer.

This will be something new for most doctors. It seems likely that most doctors haven't really grasped this fundamental feature of NPfIT yet. It underlines the need, right the way through the programme, for clinical engagement.

There is another feature of NHS-CRS that points to the need for doctors, nurses and other clinical professionals to be very involved with the project in its early stages. This is an area that the LSPs call 'clinical content'. You see, the reality is that the NHS has bought a very expensive software toolkit, but when the software is delivered it probably won't contain any clinical content. Start with a simple example – patient information leaflets. When Hilda Rawthorpe visits her consultant in outpatients and gets given a diagnosis of type 2 diabetes, one of the features of NHS-CRS will be the ability for the consultant to enter a diagnosis code, and for the computer to oblige by printing out a useful leaflet for Hilda, in any one of seven languages, explaining all about diabetes. But who is going to write that leaflet? The LSPs won't. They are not medical specialists. Besides, if they did, for example, commission the content from someone who was a specialist, how could they be sure it was accurate? They might be exposed to litigation from a patient who took the advice in the leaflet and suffered an adverse event. No, the LSPs are likely to be very firm on this point. Clinical content is a matter for clinicians. Specifically it is a matter for NHS clinicians. They will deliver the application that will allow the leaflets to be printed, but they will not author them.

Out of interest, how many patient advice leaflets do you imagine the NHS will need? Printed leaflets might be given to patients in A&E, outpatients, on discharge from hospital, in the community, at GP clinics. There may be around 3000 leaflets needed.

Take another example – assessment forms. An assessment form appears on the screen when a doctor, or a nurse, or another health professional needs to examine a patient. Obviously these forms have to be specific to the particular assessment that the patient needs. An assessment for cataracts in the eye will be wholly different to an assessment for arthritis in the foot. They are complicated things, these assessment forms. If a nurse measures Jimmy's height and weight for an assessment form, then you probably wouldn't want to have to enter that data again on a second form. The next time you call up a form that would normally ask for Jimmy's height and weight you might want those fields to be prepopulated with the data that the nurse entered last time. But then again, you might not. If Jimmy is losing weight, or if he is a child who is growing fast, then you might prefer to add this each time. Isn't this complicated?

Some assessments will collect a set of information and generate a score. An example of these is an assessment of the risk that a patient will develop bed sores. Some assessments might collect historic data, but how much weight do you give that data? If you ask patients if they are allergic to penicillin, for example, some patients will answer yes even if they don't have the allergy. But if you have stored that response in a database record that is called 'allergic to penicillin', in a data field that will need to be coded to reflect this, then this allergy might appear on the patient record with as much weight and authority as it would have if it had emerged from a clinical finding. Is that what you want to happen?

LSPs are likely to treat assessment forms in the same way that they would treat patient advice leaflets; they will leave the content authorship all up to the NHS. The tools are there, the NHS and the clinicians can build their own forms. But this creates problems too. Imagine that Doctor Smith at the City Infirmary creates an assessment form that he decides to call 'Diabetes Admission Assessment Form'. That form will join a library of forms on NHS-CRS that the whole cluster will access. But who says that this is the best practice form? What if Dr Smith is a very idiosyncratic practitioner and hardly any other diabetologist in the cluster would choose to use his form? They need to create rival forms. Soon you have a library of forms that might include Dr Jones's new improved diabetes admission form, Dr Smith's diabetes admission form version 3, version 9, Dr Brown's new simplified diabetes admission assessment form. No. It won't do. You might end up with dozens, hundreds of competing forms. It won't promote best practice. So what the NHS needs is not just clinical engagement, and clinical content authorship, it is clinical governance. Someone needs to point out to the rival diabetologists that they could maybe manage with, say, two different forms. Honour would be satisfied, and good practice would hold sway.

As the programme rolls ahead, the LSPs will probably do their best to encourage clinical engagement, but it isn't necessarily easy for them. They can't identify the clinical leaders or the networks. It isn't their responsibility. This is one area where the LSPs can shrug their shoulders. Clinical content and clinical governance is the responsibility of the NHS. It is a thistle that the NHS needs to grasp pretty firmly or the new NHS-CRS will be empty of clinical content.

So how many assessment forms will we need? No one knows, but estimates vary between 5000 and 70 000. The final number is likely to be around 10 000.

Clinical content authorship will not end with leaflets and assessment forms. Integrated Care Pathways will need to be written and approved by NHS clinicians. The NHS may need well over a thousand of these. Decision support rules and alerts will need to be written and approved by NHS clinicians. The NHS will need to identify tests that can be ordered, and referrals that can be made, and examinations that can be requested from radiology or other imaging departments. The NHS will need to determine what security levels attach to every one of these items. Who has the security to order a full blood count? Who can order a chest X-ray? Who can see the results? Who can cancel an order? The LSP won't make these decisions. The NHS must do it.

Another area which will need considerable thought over the next few years is normal ranges. If Jimmy had a blood test in, say, Huddersfield and then had another when he was involved in an accident dry-slope skiing in, say, Cornwall, although the tests he had were the same, the results would be expressed against a normal range, and the normal ranges may be different. So – if you suddenly had the ability to plot on a graph all of Jimmy's lab results, and you plotted the graph of his results regardless of where these tests were performed, you may not be comparing like with like.

Why? A normal range is established in the lab where the test is performed. The range depends upon the equipment and reagents used. They will not always be the same. In a recently merged Trust, the two hospitals each kept their own pathology laboratories. So there were two haematology laboratories, and two biochemistry labs. If Jimmy had a cardiac enzyme test done in one biochemistry lab (now from the same Trust) the significance of the result (is it normal?) might depend on which of the two labs the cardiac enzymes were tested in. The LSPs will not sort this can of worms out. It will have to be resolved by clinicians. Clinical engagement then is not an optional luxury for NPfIT. It is absolutely central and fundamental.

In the end, that is the message of this book. NPfIT has the potential to be the biggest catalyst for change that the National Health Service in England has ever seen. It is a bold, far-reaching project that has the power to transform the delivery of healthcare, to overturn old processes and replace them with efficient stream-lined ways to deliver care. It has the potential to improve outcomes, to reduce mistakes, and to help build a healthier nation. But it will only do this with the consent and the support of the people who have to use it – the doctors, the nurses, the dentists, the laboratory scientists, the radiographers, the medical secretaries, the ward clerks, the physiotherapists and other therapists, the counsellors, the chaplains, the midwives and the whole mosaic of dedicated, hard-working care givers and health professionals who together make up the NHS.

It isn't a challenge for the computer teams any more.

The challenge now, is for them.

Interview with Frank Burns

January 2002

In September 1998 a document was released on the NHS which would outline a vision of how Information Management and Technology (IM&T), if properly implemented and resourced, would change for the better the way healthcare is delivered. The document was *Information for Health* and its author was Mr Frank Burns CBE, the Chief Executive of Wirral Hospitals NHS Trust.

Four years on, and three years before the major milestones identified in that document as a measurement of progress were expected to be delivered, I interviewed the author to assess his views on progress to date.

Q: Do you think that setting targets in Information for Health was a 'good thing to do?'
Yes. If we had simply written a document, a vision of where we wanted to go, it would just have been that – a document. I still believe we were right to put in place a mechanism for measuring our progress towards this vision.

Q: We all acknowledge that the NHS has been very slow to embrace IM&T, and yet there are examples of where this is not the case, and it is usually where the Chief Executive has been the driving force. What evidence did you need to see that enabled you to actively support these IT systems in your hospital?
Look at any successful EPR sites. They all have buy-in from the top, but more importantly, there is always a good bunch of senior clinical staff and quality IT staff. If you can get that mixture right in a particular location and they can deliver some sustainable local advantage from investment in IT, then the Chief Executive will be interested. In my case, I didn't decide to invest in the EPR system we ultimately developed. That decision had been taken before I took up the post. And that decision had been made because of the enthusiasm of the clinical and IT staff. My only decision was that this was not going to be another NHS IT failure that was going to drag me down!

I came to this Trust when that decision to invest considerable amounts of money in the IT system had been made when similar large IT projects were going up in smoke all around the country. I learned from others' mistakes and so I decided it needed my personal attention and interest if it was to succeed.

It was more about me doing my job as a Chief Executive properly i.e. to protect public investment on a considerable scale. It was more that that initiated my interest and involvement at the beginning rather than any knowledge or skills I brought to the party at the time.

Q: So what was the driver behind Wirral's decision to invest what you described as a considerable amount of resource into IT, at a time when similar projects were going pear-shaped?
Let's be very clear about this. You don't buy clinical information systems to save

money. They are an investment in the same way a CT scanner is. They are part of the clinical infrastructure of the organisation. You can't possibly impose cost reduction burdens on IT that you wouldn't impose on any other section of the business. These systems will deliver whatever savings they are capable of delivering but they are not an efficiency measure, they are part of the clinical infrastructure of the organisation – a clinical tool. Its like an operating theatre. You wouldn't *not* buy an operating theatre because it doesn't save you money.

Q: Would you advocate a National EPR Solution?
I do get nervous that there are people far away from the reality of implementing the strategy and very far away from the culture in the NHS who have this notion that they can simply contract at a national level, for a national solution. I am sure there are still people who think that.

I personally think it would be a disaster if ever such an approach were attempted.

Integrating healthcare records over the lifetime of an individual, through a whole series of ill-health events, involving a combination of agencies and dozens of different professionals is complex and requires excellent technical solutions and vast degrees of cultural and organisational change.

To suggest you can build that and roll it out in the same way that you would roll out a supermarket check-out system displays, to me, incredible naivety that would make you seriously concerned about their understanding of the complexity of healthcare.

My great concern is that any national solution would have to be watered down to make it nationally acceptable, and, for instance, they would drop out the prescribing component of any national EPR solution because the prescribing component is so culturally difficult. You have to work at this with the local community, so my worry would be the higher the level of centralisation the lower the spec. So it would be a complete shell, a national e-mail system instead of what was intended.

Q: In the Audit Commission's recent report 'A Spoonful of Sugar' they reinforce the importance of the inclusion of Electronic Prescribing in the EPR mandatory targets, but one of their recommendations is a national prescribing solution. Does that worry you?
Let us firstly separate the specification of a national solution from the provision of a national solution.

I have no problems with a national specification and indeed Electronic Prescribing lends itself nicely to such an approach. But then the process of selecting the modules and the order of their implementation should be locally determined. Project Management and procurement should be a local decision but I have no problems with a national core specification.

Electronic Prescribing was included in the mandated targets because of its ability to significantly reduce potential harm.

What people seem to forget is that there are principally two ways to do harm during the delivery of healthcare. Through surgery and through medicines. The giving of medicines in the NHS is not a peripheral process, almost every patient receives medication in one form or another and so the potential to do harm is great. That potential is greatly increased today with the complexity of drug regimes currently used and so now the giving of medicines should be considered as dangerous as surgery.

But it is not just in the reduction of risk that electronic prescribing brings benefit, but also in helping identify what works and what doesn't. Supporting clinical processes is one aim of IfH. The secondary use of such information will then enable us to decide what works and what doesn't and there was never a more important time to assess the efficacy of effort.

Q: So do you think this would enable us to reduce the bureaucracy of procurement?
Yes, if we agree a national core spec and accreditation of systems. On two levels. You need innovation and creation and you will stifle that if you only impose national solutions. I would say that if you are procuring against a nationally defined milestone or target, you should procure against accredited systems. But if you are procuring ahead of them then you should be free to innovate.

One of the mistakes we made with the strategy was the notion of 'levels' of EPR, in that it implies levels of difficulty. If a Trust is starting from scratch, then level 3 implies a considerable degree of difficulty. I understand where the model came from and it was useful in identifying the notion of a logical sequence of events, but it implies degrees of difficulty. A 'level 3' EPR is the very least we should expect our NHS Trusts to have. It is fundamental basic functionality. In hindsight we should have called it Basic EPR. So 'level 3' delivers Basic EPR, followed by Intermediate and finally Advanced.

The term 'EPR' also implies the sole objective is to produce an electronic version of the paper record, whereas the real intention is to support clinicians with IT. That is where the real benefits lie. What may have been a better term is Electronic Patient Care Management systems or Patient Care Information Systems.

Q: What other obstacles are there to implementing IfH?
A major obstacle has been the diversion of additional funds, which had been intended for the implementation of IFH. The fact that this has been allowed to happen poses questions as to the desire of Chief Executives to deliver IfH and casts equal doubt over the part of the Department of Health and Ministers.

We should also not allow ourselves to be diverted from the aims of IfH with uncoordinated Department of Health additions to the priorities. These are often piecemeal and stand-alone solutions including NHS Direct, booked admissions, Emergency EHR for example.

Taking the last example, the Emergency EHR has been promoted in importance to the locally derived EHRs (fed by the EPRs). This inversion of importance is seriously flawed in that the Emergency EHR (in the absence of the local EHR and EPRs) will be of actual benefit to relatively few patients. We have clearly defined what we have to do, let us give the suppliers and the NHS community a stable target and not constantly chop and change it.

Q: Part of your solution to deliver IfH was the disbanding of the Information Management Group and the establishment of a new structure – the Information Policy Unit (IPU) and the Information Authority. Has this worked as you envisaged?
In some ways there is an apparent lack of leadership. This may be a perception but that perception may be due to the inability of the IA and the IPU to agree their respective roles.

The original strategy quite clearly placed upon the IA the responsibility for co-ordinating and leading national implementation. The IPU was intended to be a small high powered clique operating within the policy side of the DH to ensure

IfH implications of new policy were properly considered and fed through to the IA as necessary. There is no visible high profile champion for this strategy at national level and the NHS needs one.

Q: As you stated earlier, the NHS is in a constant state of reorganisation. We are now facing another with the removal of the Regional Offices (who were central to your IfH implementation process) and the Health Authorities to be replaced with the Strategic Health Authorities. Who now owns the IfH implementation?
I refer back to IfH. It called for the stripping out of unnecessary processes at Regional and National levels. If Strategic Health Authorities are to be trusted with a total NHS spend of billions of pounds, then surely they can be trusted to manage all the IfH investments without reference to Regions, Department of Health or the Treasury. But someone within that new organisation should be charged with ensuring the momentum for IfH does not falter.

Whilst it is reasonable that IfH implementation is performance-managed and coordinated at SHA level (collaborative procurements, etc.), it would be a huge mistake to try to force local clinical communities into single SHA-wide projects. SHAs are strategic bureaucracies, they are not natural clinical communities and are too remote to deliver locally owned solutions.'

Q: We still have (almost) four years in which to deliver the major milestones in your strategy. What needs to be done in that time to ensure these targets are met?
There needs to be a reinforcement of the political will to make this happen. The target dates must be reinforced. We need to see an urgent reduction in bureaucracy as outlined before.

The funding issues must be resolved and the promises of extra resources must materialise, fulfilling the sums notified in advance. As author of IfH, I support the ring-fencing of monies for the implementation of IfH. As a Chief Executive I am less enthusiastic for it. However, as a Chief Executive I would conclude that if the deliverables are at the core of the modernising of services, and they are profoundly important in improving clinical outcome, and if they are fundamental to the implementation of NSFs, then the implementation of *Information for Health* must be a very high priority to Chief Executives. Therefore, some sort of ring-fencing or earmarking is useful.

Q: Finally, given your time again, would you do anything differently?
I still believe the strategy has fulfilled its purpose – in defining a vision with clearly defined measurable markers of progress. It is rewarding to see a common IT goal for all the NHS and even if it takes ten years instead of seven it is like putting the plumbing in: once it is in there it will serve its purpose.

There has always been a degree of reconceptualising, especially at the academic end of interest. But we shouldn't lose sight of the difficulties that have to be overcome for this to be a success. It is actually very difficult to do, and anyone who thinks otherwise has yet to do it. I hope we can stop reconceptualising and all get down to putting these basic building blocks in place. We need basic clinical systems in place at the GP end of the service and in our hospitals, and these local implementations of IfH will support local agendas. Let us not focus on standalone projects such as the Emergency EHR, but rather put more effort into ensuring the basic building blocks are in place such as the local community EHR. These will then feed these national projects.

The document never attempted to define how IfH should be delivered (in technical terms) and I believe it has stood the test of time and is just as relevant to the NHS in 2002 as it was in 1998.

I still believe that its fundamental principles are a 'no-brainer' and there is still time for it to be delivered in a way which will fundamentally improve the delivery of clinical care, which was after all its primary objective.

An interview with Sir John Pattison

Sir John Pattison was seen as the lead civil servant for the new national programme which would become NPfIT.

At the time of this interview (2002), there had been relatively little information released about this new national IT programme. It hadn't even been decided how many PSPs there should be. (PSPs? Don't you meant LSPs? No – they were originally called Prime Service Providers and we didn't know if there were going to be 5, 10 or 28 of these creatures.)

2002!

It is amazing just how far we have come in such a short time isn't it?

There is value in revisiting the interview given to the author at that time and in the light of what we now know.

Q: Sir John, since the early nineties, specific targets have been set for IT in the NHS, but we have also had a history of consistent slippage. Why should the current targets be any different and will we be sitting here in five years explaining why these latest targets have been missed?

We must turn around the current mindset that missing targets is acceptable.

Previous targets have slipped due to issues around leadership (or lack of), timeliness and resources. I am confident that the targets this time round will be achieved because we have addressed these three issues head on. Let's take a look at each of these issues in turn . . .

Leadership

This has been tackled in three ways. Firstly a Ministerial Task Force was established to ensure the focus on the targets has commitment from the heart of government. In addition, a Department of Health individual (myself) has been identified and thirdly a national Director General of IT will soon be appointed.

History shows us that whilst this strategy for NHS IT has been built on the previous strategies (in fact many of the targets are updated and redefined historical targets), it has often been left to the enthusiasm of individuals in the NHS to ensure these strategies have succeeded.

This has resulted in pockets of excellence throughout the NHS but not the broad acceptance throughout the NHS that is required. By providing very clear national leadership, the targets will become fundamental building blocks to modernising the way healthcare is delivered.

Timeliness

We have a history of enthusiasts attempting to move forward the informatics agenda but many others have been apathetic at best. However, there is now in society a groundswell of expectation that the NHS should benefit from technology in the way that certain elements of society have benefited. It is now expected by healthcare professionals that they should have access in their work to basic technology that they have easy access to in their home.

We now find that generally the culture of our society is more electronically enabled – whether it is online banking or shopping.

Q: You are not suggesting that managing the delivery of healthcare is as simple as managing a bank account or your weekly shop?
No. Healthcare is a very complex process or series of complex processes and anyone who thinks layering a computer on top of those complex processes will achieve the desired effect is mistaken. However, there are fundamental data flows underpinning the more complex clinical activities, which can be aided by IT. The underlying science of what we are proposing in the IT programme of work is actually quite ordinary. However, the scale of what we are proposing is extraordinary. In order to ensure it happens, we have addressed the third barrier:

Resources

In the past we have failed to protect additional budget that was intended to push forward the information and technology agenda. Any additional hard fought for money, which was 'loosely' identified for IM&T, by earmarking or hypothecation, was very susceptible to being raided for more short-term use. Chief executives appreciated the need for long-term investment in information, but with immediate pressures on their budgets understandably they often fell to that temptation.

And now to the new programme of work. There is still some confusion as to the thinking behind the 'Greek Temple' programme of work taking the three pillars: prescribing, health records and online booking. This is a very false demarcation of work and by fragmenting it up in this way there will be very fragmented solutions when they are in reality dependent upon each other.

An elephant is an elephant however you assemble it. As long as the end vision is shared, it is sensible to focus on the critical individual components that make up the entire beast. So, we have broken down the overall programme into bite-sized components, which allows us to focus on each of them individually. The end objective is a complete solution, but during its development, the focus has to be on smaller components. These are:

Infrastructure

The least 'exciting', but nonetheless fundamental to the success of all elements, is the work needed to put the infrastructure in place. The health service and the people who work in it and have cause to use it, should not have to 'make do' with inferior technology that other elements of society readily take for granted.

We want to avoid giving those people less IT capability than their children receive at primary school, with high-speed networks now being made available to all schools and colleges. That means we should not have to accept a network that is slow and incapable of supporting the kind of fast data flows that clinicians will need. The infrastructure elements are essential building blocks to achieve the ultimate objective.

Data and IT standards are essential if we are to allow flexibility in the delivery of clinical solutions. Interoperability between different components can only be achieved if dogmatic national technical standards are developed and complied with. The accreditation process will enable the implementation of these nationally agreed standards.

Electronic record

Providing a shared electronic record is a fundamental requirement of delivering a modern integrated healthcare service. This element of the Programme of Work is now expressed as the Integrated Care Record Service and will be responsible for the delivery of just that. As you know, the biggest gains to be made are through using technology to support a patient through his/her care pathways and there are now real opportunities offered by modern technology to enable this to happen more efficiently.

Online booking

Whilst acknowledging that healthcare is complex and the data flows are not as simple as those required for online banking or booking plane tickets, there are nonetheless real clinical benefits to be gained from computerising the basic patient journey data flows. People are now expecting and demanding better access to services. Online booking is the start, to remove unnecessary anxiety by reducing waiting times and then making the patient's journey through the healthcare system more visible. But this is just the start. There is little point in simply computerising the appointment process without making available all the relevant information to those charged with their care. Online booking together with the Integrated Care Record Service will enable more efficient service to be delivered to the patient.

Electronic prescribing

This pillar of work is the Electronic Transmission of Prescriptions between GP, community pharmacies and the Prescribing Pricing Authority (PPA). We now have three pilots to test the issues around the secure electronic transfer of prescriptions. We will focus on those four areas and together with the delivery of organisational integrated clinical systems (or EPRs) we can create a more effective and efficient experience for the patients.

Q: So, are the previously called EPR – 'organisational-based' systems – still valid along with their targets?
Yes. We still expect Trusts to be prescribing electronically, using integrated clinical systems with the outputs from them contributing to the Integrated Care Record. We still expect all Trusts to have actively implemented basic elements and functionality of electronic records by December 2005.

Q: There are major concerns in the supplier industry around the proposed changes in the way underpinning systems for all the above are procured. The recent announcements have resulted in a degree of 'planning blight' with Trusts playing the waiting game until the new strategy becomes clearer. Are we not going to have a problem like the railway industry which is that by the time the promised modernisation monies appeared, the rolling stock manufacturers had disappeared – so they had the investment but have to go abroad to buy our trains! How do we manage that gap?
I am aware of the situation in the supplier industry and do not want the NHS to go on hold with their planning. The new processes are long overdue – everyone acknowledges the present procurement process is untenable. However, doing nothing is not an option and I am aware that there are a number of large procurements underway. It is not our intention to obstruct or prevent such procurements, but it is essential that all existing and planned procurements are

compatible with the national strategy. To this end there will be a review of those already underway.

Q: As I understand it, you are introducing a new 'tier' in the procurement i.e. the PSPs (Prime Service Providers) who will be contracted by Strategic Health Authorities (StHAs) to deliver the systems required and identified by local Trusts. Is this not simply adding an expensive additional layer on an already bureaucratic process?
We are removing the intense bureaucracy at the Trust level. The effort currently required to identify a specification, a business case and go through the selection process is onerous and is undertaken by healthcare staff in addition to their already busy lives. It is envisaged that the contract negotiations will be taken away for that level and undertaken between PSPs and Strategic Health Authorities.

Q: But couldn't the existing process be improved simply by a) developing national business cases b) ring-fenced monies and c) accreditation?
There is an issue of capability. What we are proposing is extraordinary in scale and it is precisely the scale of the programme that requires this additional layer. It is needed to ensure not only that the technology solutions are available and accredited, but to underpin those implementations with comprehensive change management. We know that some enthusiasts will forge ahead whatever model is adopted, but it is the generality that require more support and facilitation. The traditional procurement model is not designed to do this and the scale of what we are proposing needs this extra change management facilitation layer.

Q: But by taking the selection of solutions up to the Strategic Health Authority, are you not moving choice further away from the sharp end?
It is imperative that we get clinical buy-in to the solutions selected. The Strategic Health Authorities will not undertake the selection process in isolation but will have to engage with the clinical users at the Trust. This model is already being used through local collaborative procurement schemes. Many Trusts in London are beginning to think at a level above the single Trust and there are economies of scale to be had through such collaborations. For example the BlackBerd initiative in Birmingham and at North Essex at the Paddington Basin.

Traditional isolated procurements are perceived as not being efficient and as the boundaries between organisations become more blurred, so conformity of systems is becoming essential.

In some areas, such as Lambeth, Southwark and Lewisham, all General Practitioners have now agreed to use the same GP system. That has happened naturally and is not a response to a central diktat or target.

Q: History has shown us the great difficulty we have in gaining consensus from clinical groups on informatics issues. How are you going to get the various clinical groups to agree a national specification for these complex and comprehensive clinical systems?
The clinical system information needs of a physician are different to those of a surgeon, a nurse or a physiotherapist. We have not attempted to agree a national specification at a detailed level but have sought agreement for the core components of the systems.

It is these core specifications that each supplier will be accredited against and once a product has been accredited, it would be available through a call-off contract managed by the PSP.

Q: As I understand it, most contracts will be PSP to StHA with PSPs gathering together a number of suppliers with accredited product sets to be made available through call-off contracts. This could mean that every supplier needs to have a relationship with all the PSPs. Is this not simply moving the bureaucracy up a level?
Its not even as simple as that! There is a large legacy to deal with – systems that have been successfully implemented and used for years. These will not be immediately replaced and any arrangement with a PSP will have to allow for such existing applications. There will also have to be Service Level Agreements with the suppliers of national services such as the NHS network.

Q: You have indicated that you are impressed with the work done in Scotland. Do you see their model as one that could be replicated in England?
There has been some very good central direction given and followed in Scotland, but again it's a question of scale. What we are doing is on an extraordinary scale, and you have to remember that Scotland is the size of one of our old Regions. We do not have the evidence that we could achieve the same results in a country 10 times larger. There are elements of the programme that will be better delivered through central procurements, others through local procurements (through the StHA) following central core specification. It is important that we clearly identify and articulate the scope of what is and what isn't core. This work is underway and will be delivered in the coming months.

Q: Finally Sir John, whilst we all acknowledge there had to be change, and even assuming we are all enthusiasts for the vision, what evidence is there that the model you propose will work?
As you say doing nothing is not an option. The direction in Delivering the NHS Plan is to devolve responsibility and resources to the frontline. However, the evidence from successful large scale and corporate deployment and use of IT indicates that we must move away from separate systems based around organisations. National standards aim to ensure interoperability and national applications aim to ensure a consistent service. Finally, we need to protect and target the significant new funding to ensure that we can deliver our priorities, and referring back to your opening question, to ensure that we meet our core targets.

Appendix 3

Common abbreviations and acronyms

A&C	Administrative & Clerical
A&E	Accident & Emergency
ABI	Area-Based Initiative
ABM	Activity-Based Management
ABPI	Association of the British Pharmaceutical Industry
AC	Audit Commission
ACAC	Area Clinical Audit Committee
ACAS	Advisory, Conciliation & Arbitration Service
ACHC	Association of Community Health Councils
ACHCEW	Association of Community Health Councils in England & Wales
ACIG	Academy of Medical Royal Colleges Information Group
ACMT	Advisory Committee on Medical Training
ADC	Automatic Data Capture
ADP	Automatic Data Processing
ADR	Adverse Drug Reaction
AHP	Allied Health Professional
AICU	Adult Intensive Care Unit
AIM	Advanced Informatics in Medicine
AIMS	Association for Improvements in Maternity Services
ALERT	Acute Life-threatening Events Recognition and Treatment
ALOS	Average Length of Stay
AMRC	Academy of Medical Royal Colleges
APH	Association of Public Health
APIR	Assessment, Planning, Implementation and Review
AQH	Association for Quality in Healthcare
ASSIST	Association for Information Management and Technology Staff in the NHS
ASP	Application Service Provider
ATTRACT	Ask Trip to Rapidly Alleviate Confused Thoughts
AVG	Ambulatory Visit Group
BAMM	British Association of Medical Managers
BC	Block Contracting
BGM	Board General Manager
BIR	British Institute of Radiology
BIS	Business Intelligence System
BMA	British Medical Association
BMIS	British Medical Informatics Society
BMJ	*British Medical Journal*
BNF	British National Formulary
BPC	British Pharmaceutical Codex

BPL	Blood Products Laboratory
BTS	Blood Transfusion Service
CASP	Critical Appraisal Skills Programme
CASPE	Clinical Accountability Service Planning and Evaluation Specialist Healthcare Training Group
CAT	Critically Appraised Topic
CCE	Completed Consultant Episode
CCEPP	Cochrane Collaboration on Effective Professional Practice
CCP	Community Care Plans
CCT	Compulsory Competitive Tendency
CDM	Chronic Disease Management
CG	Clinical Governance
CHC	Community Health Council
CHD	Coronary Heart Disease
CHDGP	Connection of Health Data and General Practice
CHI	Commission for Health Improvement (now the Healthcare Commission)
CHIME	Centre for Health Informatics in Medical Education
CHIQ	Centre for Health Information Quality
CHMU	Central Health Monitoring Unit
CHOU	Central Health Outcomes Unit
CIC	Common Information Core
CIS	Clinical Information System
CLIB	Cochrane Library
CLIMP	Clinical Information Management Programme
CME	Continuing Medical Education
CMMS	Case Mix Management System
CMO	Chief Medical Officer/Clinical Medical Officer
CNO	Chief Nursing Officer
CNS	Clinical Nurse Specialist
CNST	Clinical Negligence Scheme for Trusts
COPC	Community-Oriented Primary Care
COPD	Chronic Obstructive Pulmonary Disease
COSHH	Control of Substances Hazardous to Health
CPA	Care Programme Approach
CPC	Cost Per Case
CPD	Continuing Professional Development
CPEP	Clinical Practice Evaluation Programme
CRAG	Clinical Research and Audit Group (Scotland)
CRD	Centre for Reviews and Dissemination
CSAG	Clinical Standards Advisory Group
CSASHS	Common Services Agency for the Scottish Health Service
DGH	District General Hospital
DHA	District Health Authority
DICE	Disseminating Information on Clinical Effectiveness
DMC	District Medical Committee
DoH	Department of Health
DPT	District Planning Team
DQB	Data Quality Project
DRG	Diagnosis-Related Group

DSU	Day Surgery Unit
EBL	Evidence-Based Learning
EBM	Evidence-Based Medicine
EBP	Evidence-Based Practice
EFMI	European Federation for Medical Informatics
E-GIF/E-GIF	Electronic Government Interoperability Framework
EHO	Environmental Health Officer
EHR	Electronic Health Record
EMR	Electronic Medical Record
EMS	Emergency Medical Services
ENP	Emergency Nurse Practitioner
ENT	Ear, Nose & Throat
EPACT	Electronic Prescribing Analysis and Costing
EPR	Electronic Patient Record
EQUIP	Effectiveness and Quality in Practice Group
ERDIP	Electronic Record Development and Implementation Programme
ETPC	Education and Training Programme in Informatics Management and Technology for Clinicians
FCE	Finished Consultant Episode
FHS	Family Health Services
FHSA	Family Health Services Authority
FHSCU	Family Health Services Computer Unit
FM	Facilities Management
FP	Family Physician
GATT	General Agreement on Tariff & Trade
GENECIS	General Clinical Information System
GMC	General Medical Council
GMP	General Medical Practitioner
GMS	General Medical Services
GP	General Practitioner
GPASS	General Practice Administration System (Scotland)
GPC	General Practitioners Committee
GPS	General Pharmaceutical Services
HA	Health Authority
HAA	Hospital Activity Analysis/Health Action Area
HAAC	Health Action Area Coordinator
HAC	Health Advisory Committee
HAS	Health Advisory Service
HAZ	Health Action Zones
HB	Health Board
HBG	Health Benefit Group
HC	Health Circular/Health Centre
HCEU	Healthcare Evaluation Unit
HCHS	Hospital & Community Health Services
HELMIS	Health Management Information Service
HES	Hospital Episode Statistics
HIG	Health Implementation Group
HIMP	Health Improvement and Modernisation Programme
HIP	Health Improvement Programme

HIS	Health Informatics Service
HISS	Hospital Information Support Systems
HMB	Health Modernisation Board
HMR	Hospital Medical Record
HR	Human Resources
HRG	Healthcare Resource Group
HSG	Health Service Guidance
HSI	Health Service Indicator
HSJ	Health Service Journal
HTA	Health Technology Assessment
HTM	High Technology Medicine
ICD	International Classification of Disease
ICP	Integrated Care Pathway
ICRS	Integrated Care Records Service
ICWS	Integrated Clinical Workstation
IfH	*Information for Health*
IFM	Information for the Management of Healthcare
IHRIM	Institute of Health Record Information and Management
IHSM	Institute of Health Services Management
IIP	Investors In People
IM&T	Information Management and Technology
IPA	Indicative Prescribing Amount
IPR	Individual Performance Review
IR	Independent Review
IRP	Independent Review Panel
JCC	Joint Consultative Committee
JEIS-ERDIP	Information Sharing Project With Social Services
JFC	Joint Formulary Committee
LA	Local Authority
LAPIS	Locality and Practice Information
LDP	Local Development Plan
LDS	Local Development Scheme
LHG	Local Health Group
LHP	Local Health Partnerships
LIS	Local Implementation Strategies
LMC	Local Medical Committee
LMS	Licentiate of Medicine and Surgery
LOS	Length of Stay
LSP	Local Strategic Partnerships
LSP	Local Service Providers
LTM	Learning to Manage Health Information
MAC	Medical Advisory Committee
MAGG	Multidisciplinary Audit Advisory Group
MC	Medicines Commission
MCA	Medical Control Agency
MCQ	Multiple Choice Questions
MD	Medicine Doctor (Doctor of Medicine)
MDA	Medical Devices Agency
MEC	Management Education for Clinicians

MIG	Medical Information Group
MLSO	Medical Laboratory Scientific Officer
MPC	Medical Practices Committee
MRO	Medical Records Officer
NAO	National Audit Office
NASP	National Application Service Provider
NBTS	National Blood Transfusion Service
NCCA	National Centre for Clinical Audit
NCMO	National Case Mix Office
NCRS	National Care Records Service
NeLH	National electronic Library for Health
NHS	National Health Service
NHS-CRS	NHS Care Records Service
NHSIA	National Health Service Information Authority
NHSIMC	National Health Service Information Centre
NHSiS	NHS in Scotland
NHSLA	National Health Service Litigation Authority
NHST	National Health Service Trust
NHSTF	National Health Service Trust Federation
NICE	National Institute for Clinical Excellence
NISP	National Infrastructure Service Provider
NMAC	National Medical Advisory Committee
NMIS	Nurse Management Information System
NPfIT	National Programme for Information Technology
NPSA	National Patient Safety Agency
NPT	Near-Patient Testing
NRE	Non-Recurring Expenditure
NSF	National Service Framework
OAT	Out of Area Treatment
OATS	Out of Area Treatments
OCS	Order Communications System
OCS/RR	Order Communications (Systems)/Results Reporting
OD	Organisational Development
OH	Occupational Health
OP	Outpatient
OPD	Outpatient Department
OR	Operation Research
PACE	Purchasing Authority Chief Executives
PACS	Picture Archiving and Communication System
PACT	Prescription Analysis and Cost
PAF	Performance Assessment Framework
PALS	Patients Advice and Liaison Services
PAM	Profession Allied to Medicine
PAS	Patient Administrative System
PCAG	Primary Care Audit Group
PCCG	Primary Care Coordinating Group
PCG	Primary Care Group
PCT	Primary Care Trust
PDA	Personal Digital Assistant

PFC	Patient-Focused Care
PGCME	Postgraduate and Continuing Medical Education
PH	Public Health
PHA	Public Health Alliance
PHC	Primary Healthcare
PHCDS	Public Health Common Data Set
PHCSG	Primary Health Care Specialist Group
PHCT	Primary Health Care Team
PHL	Public Health Laboratory
PHLS	Public Health Laboratory Service
PHPU	Public Health Policy Unit
PHRU	Public Health Resource Unit
PHSS	Personal Health Summary System
PI	Performance Indicator
PMS	Primary Medical Services
POM	Prescription Only Medicines
PPA	Prescription Pricing Authority
PRD	Performance Review and Development
PRIMIS	Primary Care Information Services
PRINCE	Projects in Controlled Environments
PSM	Professions Supplementary to Medicine
PSP	Primary Service Provider – former name for LSP
PSNC	Pharmaceutical Services Negotiating Committee
QA	Quality Assurance
QAA	Quality Assurance Authority
QALY	Quality Adjusted Life Year
QMAS	Quality Management and Analysis Service
QUANGO	Quasi-autonomous Non-governmental Organisation
R&D	Research & Development
RAWP	Resource Allocation Working Party
RDA	Recommended Daily Allowance
RDO	Regional Development Organisation
RM	Resource Management
RMI	Resource Management Initiative
RMN	Registered Mental Nurse
RMO	Resident Medical Officer
RO	Regional Office
RR	Relative Risk
RSM	Royal Society of Medicine
SAGNIS	Strategic Advisory Group for Nursing Information Systems
SGHT	Standing Group On Health Technology
SHA	Strategic Health Authority
SLA	Service Level Agreement
SMAC	Standing Medical Advisory Committee
SMART	Specific, Measurable, Achievable (or Attainable), Realistic and Timely
SODoH	Scottish Department of Health
SOHHD	Scottish Home Office and Health Department
SPA	Scottish Prescribing Analysis
SUS	Secondary Uses Service

TRIP	Turning Research Into Practice
UKCC	United Kingdom Central Council for Nursing, Midwifery and Health Visiting (now the Nursing and Midwifery Council)
UMT	Unit of Medical Time
WAHAT	Welsh Association of Health Authorities and Trusts
WFP	*Working For Patients*
WHO	World Health Organization
WTI	Waiting Time Initiative

Useful website addresses

The following links were checked in December 2004. They will be constantly updated online at www.thebiggestcomputerprogrammeintheworldever.com.

NPfIT

NPfIT: www.npfit.nhs.uk
Choose and Book: www.chooseandbook.nhs.uk
BT: www.bt.com
Accenture: www.Accenture.co.uk
Fujitsu: http://uk.fujitsu.com/
CSC: http://csc.co.uk
iSOFT PLC: www.isoftplc.com
IDX: http://idx.com
Atos Origin: www.atosorigin.co.uk/

Clinical audit

Clinical Governance Resource and Development Unit, University of Leicester:
   www.le.ac.uk/cgrdu
National Institute for Clinical Excellence: www.nice.org.uk
Royal Pharmaceutical Society of Great Britain Clinical Audit Unit: www.rpsgb.org.uk/
   audhome.htm

Clinical governance

British Journal of Clinical Governance: www.mcb.co.uk/bjcg.htm
Clinical Governance in the London Region: www.doh.gov.uk/ntro/share.htm
The Clinical Governance Resource and Development Unit, University of Leicester:
   www.le.ac.uk/cgrdu/
NHS Information Authority: www.nhsia.nhs.uk/def/home.asp?
PRODIGY: www.prodigy.nhs.uk/
Royal College of Psychiatrists' Research Unit (CRU): www.rcpsych.ac.uk/cru/
   cru_home.htm
Wisdom: www.wisdomnet.co.uk/default.asp

Evidence-based practice

ACP Journal Club: www.acponline.org/journals/acpjc/jcmenu.htm
Bandolier: www.jr2.ox.ac.uk:80/bandolier/
Centre for Evidence-Based Child Health: www.ich.ucl.ac.uk/ich/html/academicunits/
   paed_epid/cebch/
Centre for Evidence-Based Medicine: http://cebm.jr2.ox.ac.uk/

Centre for Evidence-Based Mental Health: www.cebmh.com
Centre for Evidence-Based Nursing: www.york.ac.uk/healthsciences/centres/
    evidence/cebn.htm
Centre for Reviews and Dissemination (CRD): www.york.ac.uk/inst/crd/
    welcome.htm
Centres for Health Evidence.net: www.cche.net/
Cochrane Collaboration: www.cochrane.org/index0.htm
Cochrane Database of Systematic Reviews: www.cochrane.org/cochrane/revabstr/
    mainindex.htm
CASP (Critical Appraisal Skills Programme): www.phru.nhs.uk/casp/casp.htm
MedConnect: http://medconnect.com/
Netting the Evidence: A ScHARR introduction to evidence-based practice on the
    Internet: www.shef.ac.uk/scharr/ir/netting/
NHS Centre for Reviews and Dissemination: www.york.ac.uk/inst/crd/
Wessex Institute for Health Research and Development: www.soton.ac.uk/~wi/

General information/miscellaneous

EPR Arms: www.eprarms.com
BBC News – Health: http://news.bbc.co.uk/1/hi/health/default.stm
Behavioural Healthcare and Telehealth Resources on the Web: www.umdnj.edu/
    psyevnts/pointers.html
Campaign Against Living Miserably: www.thecalmzone.net
Charities in the UK: www.charity-choice.com/focusframe.htm
Childline: www.childline.org.uk
Diseases Explained: www.diseases-explained.com/
Doctorsworld.com: www.doctorsworld.com/
Doctors.net: www.doctors.org.uk/
Doctors.net.uk – Portal for Doctors: www.doctors.net.uk/
GPUK – The General Practitioner's mailing list: www.jiscmail.ac.uk/archives/gp-uk.html
Government Departments and Ministries of Health: European Union: www.doh.gov.uk/
    links/ec.htm
Health-News.co.uk: www.health-news.co.uk/
Healthwise: www.healthwise.org.uk
Help for Health Trust: www.hfht.org/
Internet Mental Health: www.mentalhealth.com/
KEN: www.mentalhealth.org/
Medical Defence Union: www.the-mdu.com/
Medic8.com – UK medical portal: www.medic8.com/
Medical World Search: www.mwsearch.com/
Medix UK: www.medix-uk.com/
Mental Health Infosource: www.mhsource.com/
National Library of Medicine: www.nlm.nih.gov/
National Research Register: www.update-software.com/National/
Neuropsychology Central: www.neuropsychologycentral.com/index.html
NHS Direct Online: www.nhsdirect.nhs.uk/
NursingNetUk – Database of Nursing Jobs: www.nursingnetuk.com/
Patient UK: www.patient.org.uk/
publicsecta.com: www.publicsecta.com/
Psych-Net UK: www.psychnet-uk.com/
Radcliffe Publishing: www.radcliffe-oxford.com/
Self-help Groups UK: www.ukselfhelp.info
Wellcome Trust: www.wellcome.ac.uk/

Health policy, research and publications

Agency for Healthcare Research and Quality: www.ahcpr.gov/
Audit Commission: www.audit-commission.gov.uk/
Centre for Clinical Outcomes, Research and Effectiveness (CORE):
   www.psychol.ucl.ac.uk/CORE/index.html
Centre for Health Ecomonics: www.york.ac.uk/inst/che/
Circulars on the Internet (COIN): www.doh.gov.uk/coinh.htm
Department of Health: www.dh.gov.uk/Home/fs/en
Hansard: www.parliament.the-stationery-office.co.uk/pa/cm/cmhansrd.htm
Health-related reports, inquiries, White Papers and Acts of Parliament:
   http://cwis.livjm.ac.uk/lea/info/health/heareps.htm
Health and Social Science Research Group (HSSRG), University of York:
   www.york.ac.uk/inst/iriss/hssrg.htm
Health Care Practice Research and Development Unit, University of Salford:
   www.salford.ac.uk/ihr/hcprdu/hcprdu.htm
Health Development Agency: www.hda-online.org.uk/
Health Education Board for Scotland: www.hebs.scot.nhs.uk/
House of Commons: www.parliament.uk/commons/hsecom.htm
Houses of Parliament: www.parliament.uk/hophome.htm
Institute for Health Research: www.lancs.ac.uk/users/ihr/dhrr.htm
Institute of Healthcare Management: www.ihm.org.uk/home.cfm/
Irish Department of Health and Children: www.doh.ie/
King's Fund: www.kingsfund.org.uk/
Medical Records Institute: www.medrecinst.com/
National Guidelines Clearinghouse: www.guidelines.gov/
National Institute for Clinical Excellence: www.nice.org.uk/
National Research Register: www.update-software.com/National/nrr-frame.html
New Zealand Guidelines Group: www.nzgg.org.nz/index.cfm
NHS Centre for Reviews and Dissemination: http://york.ac.uk/inst/crd/
NHS Confederation: www.nhsconfed.net/
NHS Executive: www.doh.gov.uk/nhsexec/nhseros.htm
NHS Executive Trent: www.nhsetrent.gov.uk/trentrd/rd.html
Northern Ireland Department of Health and Social Services: www.dhssni.gov.uk/
Nuffield Institute for Health: www.leeds.ac.uk/nuffield/
Nursing Research Unit: www.kcl.ac.uk/depsta/healifsci/fndnm/nru/nr-home.htm
Office for National Statistics (ONS): www.ons.gov.uk/ons_f.htm
Personal Social Services Research Unit (PSSRU): www.ukc.ac.uk/pssru/index.html
Royal College of Psychiatrists' Research Unit (CRU): www.rcpsych.ac.uk/cru/
   cru_home.htm
St George's Medical School, Health Care Evaluation Unit: www.sghms.ac.uk/phs/hceu/
   guide.htm
Sainsbury Centre for Mental Health: www.sainsburycentre.org.uk/
Scotland's Health on the Web: www.show.scot.nhs.uk
Scottish Assembly: www.scotland.gov.uk/
Scottish Development Centre for Mental Health Services: www.sdcformhs.org.uk/
Scottish Intercollegiate Guidelines Network (SIGN): www.sign.ac.uk/
The Scottish Parliament: www.scottish.parliament.uk/
Social Policy Research Unit (SPRU): www.york.ac.uk/inst/spru/
UK Official Publications on the Internet: http://offical-documents.co.uk/menu/
   ukpinf.htm
Welsh Office: www.wales.gov.uk/index_e.html

Journals and online health magazines

Academic Press (Journal of adolescence): www.academicpress.com/adolescence/
Academic Psychiatry: http://ap.psychiatryonline.org/
Advances in Psychiatric Treatment: http://apt.rcpsych.org/
American Journal of Psychiatry: http://ajp.psychiatryonline.org/
Annals of Clinical Psychiatry: www.aacp.com/annals.html
Archives of General Psychiatry: http://archpsyc.ama-assn.org/
Australasian Psychiatry: www.blacksci.co.uk/~cgilib/
   jnlpage.bin?Journal=XAUPS&File=XAUPS&Page=aims
Australia and New Zealand Journal of Psychiatry: www.blacksci.co.uk/~cgilib/
   jnlpage.bin?Journal=XANJP&File=XANJP&Page=aims
Bandolier: www.jr2.ox.ac.uk/Bandolier/
British Journal of Forensic Practice: www.pavpub.com/pavpub/journals/
   screen2.asp?Title=The+British+Journal+of+Forensic+Practice
British Journal of General Practice: www.rcgp.org.uk/publicat/journal/
British Journal of Healthcare Computing (BJHC): www.bjhc.co.uk/
British Journal of Health Care Management: www.markallengroup.com/publish/
   medical/bjhcm/index.htm
British Journal of Nursing: www.markallengroup.com/publish/medical/bjn/index.htm
British Journal of Psychiatry: http://bjp.rcpsych.org/
British Medical Informatics Society: www.bmis.org/
British Medical Journal (BMJ): http://bmj.com/
British National Formulary: http://bnf.org/
British Nursing News Online: www.nurse-nurses-nursing.com/
Child and Adolescent Psychiatry On-line: www.priory.com/psychild.htm
Clinical Evidence: www.evidence.org/index-welcome.htm
Clinical Science Online: http://cs.portlandpress.co.uk/
Doctors Guide to the Internet: www.docguide.com/
eGuidelines – clinical guidelines: www.eguidelines.co.uk/
epulse: www.epulse.co.uk/
Effective Health Care: www.york.ac.uk/inst/crd/ehcb.htm
Effectiveness Matters: www.york.ac.uk/inst/crd/em.htm
European Journal of Public Health: http://www3.oup.co.uk/jnls/list/eurpub/contents/
Evidence-Based Medicine/Best Evidence: www.bmjpg.com/data/ebm.htm
Evidence-Based Mental Health: www.psychiatry.ox.ac.uk/cebmh/journal/index2.html
Evidence-Based Nursing: www.bmjpg.com/data/ebn.htm
Forensic Psychiatry On-line: www.priory.com/forpsy.htm
German Journal of Psychiatry: www.gwdg.de/~bbandel/welcome.html
Harcourt international: www.hbuk.co.uk/
Health Economics: http://www3.interscience.wiley.com/cgi-bin/jtoc?ID=5749
Health Education Research: http://her.oupjournals.org/
Health Informatics Europe: www.hi-europe.info/
Health Informatics Journal: www.shef-ac-press.co.uk/hij.cmf
Healthcare Informatics (USA): www.healthcare-informatics.com/
Health Policy: www.elsevier.com/inca/publications/store/5/0/5/9/6/2/
   index.htt?menu=cont.cpcd
Health Policy and Planning: http://heapol.oupjournals.org/
Health Promotion International: http://heapro.oupjournals.org/
Health Service Journal (HSJ): www.hsj.co.uk/: www.ich.bmf.ac.uk/library/
   resource.htm#ebm
Hospital Bulletin: www.hospital-bulletin.co.uk/index_2.html
Inside Hospitals: www.inside-hospitals.co.uk/index_2.html

Internet Journal of Advanced Nursing Practice: www.ispub.com/journals/ijanp.htm
International Journal of Eating Disorder: www.acadeatdis.org/
International Journal of Epidemiology: http://ije.oupjournals.org/contents-by-date.0.shtml
International Journal of Health Planning and Management: http://www3.interscience.wiley.com/cgi-bin/jtoc?ID=4005
International Journal of Medical Informatics: www.elsevier.nl/inca/publications/store/5/0/6/0/4/0/
International Journal of Nursing Studies: www.elsevier.com/inca/publications/store/2/6/6/index.htt?menu=cont.cpcd
International Journal of Psychosocial Rehabilitation: www.psychosocial.com/
International Journal for Quality in Healthcare: http://www3.oup.co.uk/intqhc/contents/
International Journal of Social Psychiatry: www.ijsp.co.uk/
Internet Journal of Mental Health: www.ispub.com/journals/ijmh.htm
Irish Medical Journal: http://imj.ie/
ITIN – British Computer Society Nursing Specialist Group: www.bcsnsg.org.uk/itin/
Journal of Advanced Nursing: www.blackwell-science.com/~cgilib/jnlpage.bin?Journal=JAN&File=JAN&Page=contents
Journal of the American Academy of Child and Adolescent Psychiatry: www.aacap.org/publications/journal/index.htm
Journal of the American Medical Association: http://jama.ama-assn.org/
The Journal of Clinical Psychiatry: www.psychiatrist.com/
Journal of Community Nursing: www.jcn.co.uk/home.htm
Journal of Forensic Psychiatry: www.tandf.co.uk/journals/frameloader.html?www.tandf.co.uk/journals/routledge/09585184.html
Journal of Health Economics: www.elsevier.com/cgi-bin/cas/tree/store/jhe/cas_free/browse/browse.cgi/
Journal of Medical Ethics: http://jme.bmjjournals.com/
The Journal of Medical Internet Research: www.jmir.org/default.htm
Journal of Mental Health Policy and Economics: http://www3.interscience.wiley.com/cgi-bin/jtoc?ID=6219
Journal of Neurology, Neurosurgery and Psychiatry: http://jnnp.bmjjournals.com/
Journal of Neuropsychiatry and Clinical Neurosciences: http://neuro.psychiatryonline.org/
Journal of Nursing Management: www.blacksci.co.uk/~cgilib/jnlpage.bin?Journal=jnm&File=jnm&Page=contents
Journal of Psychiatric Practice: www.practicalpsychiatry.com/
Journal of Psychiatric Research: www.elsevier.com/inca/publications/store/2/4/1/
Journal of Psychiatry: www.medical-library.org/j_psych.htm
Journal of Psychiatry and Neuroscience: www.cma.ca/jpn/index.htm
Journal of Public Health Medicine: http://www3.oup.co.uk/jnls/list/pubmed/contents/
The Lancet: www.thelancet.com/
New England Journal of Medicine: www.nejm.org/content/index.asp
NewMeds – UK Medicines News: www.newmeds.co.uk/
New Scientist: www.newscientist.com/
Nurse Education Today: www.harcourt-international.com/journals/nedt/default.cfm?latestest.html
Nursing Standard Online: www.nursing-standard.co.uk
Nursing Times: www.nursingtimes.net/
Priory Lodge Medical Journals: www.priory.co.uk/
Psychiatric Bulletin: http://pb.rcpsych.org/
Psychiatric Care: www.stockton-press.co.uk/pc/index.html
Psychiatric Services: http://psychservices.psychiatryonline.org/

Psychiatry and the Clinical Neurosciences: www.blacksci.co.uk/~cgilib/
   jnlpage.bin?Journal=XPCN&File=XPCN&Page=aims
Psychological Medicine: www.journals.cup.org/owa_dba/owa/
   ISSUES_IN_JOURNAL?JID=PSM
Quality in Health Care: www.bmjpg.com/data/qhccur.htm; www.qualityhealthcare.com/
RCM Midwives Journal: www.midwives.co.uk/
Reuters Health Information Service: www.reutershealth.com/
Statistics in Medicine: http://www3.interscience.wiley.com/cgi-bin/jtoc?ID=2988
Telemedicine Newsletter: www.cyberhealth.bc.ca/signals.htm
Telemedicine Today: www.telemedtoday.com/
Transcultural Psychiatry: www.sagepub.co.uk/frame.html?http%3A//
   www.sagepub.co.uk/journals/details/j0183.html
Western Journal of Medicine: www.ewjm.com/
Which? Drug and Therapeutics Bulletin: www.which.net/health/dtb/main.html

Libraries and databases

ACHOO Healthcare On-line: www.achoo.com/
British Library On-line: http://opac97.bl.uk/
Best Medical Resources on the Web: www.priory.com/other.htm
BMA Library: www.library.bma.org.uk/
The British library: www.bl.uk/
The Cochrane Library: www.update-software.com/ccweb/cochrane/cdsr.htm;
   www.nhs.uk/nelh/cochrane.asp
COPAC – University Research Library Catalogue: http://copac.ac.uk/
Doctor Online: www.doctoronline.nhs.uk/
Electronic Medicines Compendium: www.emc.vhn.net/
English National Board Health Care Database: www.ulcc.ac.uk/ENB_closure.htm
Grey Literature Service – North West: http://nww.fade.nhs.uk
Health A–Z: www.healthatoz.com/
Health Libraries Group: www.la-hq.org.uk/groups/hlg/index.html
The Healthcare Libraries Unit – Oxford: http://libsun1.jr2.ox.ac.uk/
The Healthcare Libraries Unit – North West: www.lihnn.org.uk/lihnn/
   org.paneris.nwhclu.admin.Display/HCLUHome
Hyperguide to Mental Health: www.hyperguide.co.uk/mha/
Infotrieve: http://www3.infotrieve.com/medline/infotrieve/
Institute of Psychiatry Library: www.iop.kcl.ac.uk/IoP/AdminSup/Library/index.stm
ITpapers.com – The Yellow Pages of White Papers: www.itpapers.com/
Medical Matrix: www.medmatrix.org/reg/login.asp
Medline: http://ovid.bma.org.uk/; www.docnet.org.uk.drfelix/
Medscape: www.medscape.com/
Mental Health Infosource: www.mhsource.com/
Mental Health Links: www.hwic.ac.uk/links/tic/testweb/medicine/mental.htm
Mental Health Net: www.mentalhelp.net/
National electronic Library for Health: www.nelh.nhs.uk/; http://nww.nelh.nhs.uk/
National Library of Medicine: www.nlm.nih.gov/
National Research Register: www.update-software.com/nrr/
   CLIBINET.EXE?A=1&U=1001&P=10001
NHS Centre for Reviews and Dissemination: www.york.ac.uk/inst/crd/
NMAP – Resources for Nurses, Midwives and Allied Health Professions:
   www.nmap.ac.uk/
OMNI: http://omni.ac.uk/
The Online Medical Dictionary: www.graylab.ac.uk/omd/

Organising Medical Networked Information (OMNI): http://omni.ac.uk/
Patient Group Directions (PGDs): www.groupprotocols.org.uk/
Red Book Online: www.redbook.i12.com/Index.htm
Royal Society of Medicine Library Catalogue: www.roysocmed.ac.uk/librar/libcat.htm
Search Engines: www.altavista.co.uk/; www.excite.co.uk/; www.lycos.co.uk/;
    www.ukplus.co.uk/; www.google.co.uk
Social Science Information Gateway: http://sosig.esrc.bris.ac.uk/
UK National Database of Telemedicine: www.dis.port.ac.uk/ndtm/
Wellcome Institute Library: www.wellcome.ac.uk/

Media

BBC Homepage: http://news.bbc.co.uk/default.stm
Channel 4: www.channel4.com/
Channel 5: www.channel5.co.uk/
ITN: www.itn.co.uk/
ITV: www.itv.co.uk/

NHS and government health websites

ABS Online – address books (NHSnet only): http://nww.abs.nhs.uk/
ClearNET (NHSnet only): http://clearnet.mhapp.nhs.uk/
Commission for Health Improvement: www.chi.nhs.uk/
Data Protection: www.dataprotection.gov.uk
Dental Practice Board: www.dpb.nhs.uk/
Department of Health: www.doh.gov.uk/dhhome.htm
General Medical Council: www.gmc-uk.org/
eCommunity – Informatics Learning Network: www.ecommunity.nhs.uk/
Health Development Agency: www.hda-online.org.uk/
The Health Service Ombudsman (England): www.ombudsman.org.uk/
Health Technology Assessment (a national NHS R & D programme):
    www.hta.nhsweb.nhs.uk/
Information Policy Unit (IPU): www.doh.gov.uk/ipu/
ISD Online – Scotland's National Health Statistics and Information:
    www.show.scot.nhs.uk/isd/
LogisticsNet (NHSnet only): http://nww.logistics.nhs.uk
Medical Devices Agency: www.medical-devices.gov.uk/
Medicines Control Agency: www.mca.gov.uk/
National Institute of Clinical Excellence (NICE): www.nice.org.uk/
National Patients Safety Agency: www.hta.nhsweb.nhs.uk/
National Prescribing Center: www.npc.co.uk/
NHS Alliance: www.nhsalliance.org/
NHS Beacons Programme: www.modernnhs.nhs.uk/scripts/default.asp?site_id=16
NHS Careers: www.nhscareers.nhs.uk/index.html
NHS Confederation: www.nhsconfed.org/
NHS Direct: www.nhsdirect.nhs.uk/
NHS Direct Wales – Galw Iechyd Cymru: www.nhsdirect.wales.nhs.uk/
NHS Estates: www.nhsestates.gov.uk/
NHS Magazine: www.nhs.uk/nhsmagazine
NHS Plus – Occupational Health: www.nhsplus.nhs.uk
NHS Purchasing and Supply Agency (NHSnet only): http://nww.pasa.nhs.uk
nhs.uk Programme: www.nhs.uk/england/

NHS Workforce Development Confederations: www.nwlwdc.nhs.uk/
Organisation Codes Service (OCS) (NHSnet only): http://nww.nhsis.nhs.uk/ocs/
Prescribing Support Unit: www.psu.co.uk/
Prescription Pricing Authority (PPA): www.ppa.org.uk/index.htm
Health Protection Agency: www.phls.co.uk/
UK Transplant (NHSnet only): http://ntn.uktransplant.nhs.uk/
Waiting Lists and Waiting Times Data for England: www.doh.gov.uk/waitingtimes/
    index.htm

Other UK government

Audit Commission: www.audit-commission.gov.uk/
Cabinet Office: www.cabinet-office.gov.uk/
Data Protection: www.dataprotection.gov.uk/
e-Envoy (government strategy for the information age): www.e-envoy.gov.uk/
Health and Safety Executive: www.hse.gov.uk/hsehome.htm
Her Majesty's Stationery Office (HMSO): www.hmso.gov.uk/
Her Majesty's Treasury: www.hm-treasury.gov.uk/
National Audit Office: www.nao.gov.uk/
National Statistics: www.statistics.gov.uk/
Open Government Site: www.ukonline.gov.uk/
Public Record Office: www.pro.gov.uk/default.htm

Organisations and professional organisations

American Medical Association: www.ama-assn.org/
American Society of Consultant Pharmacists: www.ascp.com/
ASSIST: www.assist.org.uk/
Association of Medical Research Charities: www.amrc.org.uk/
Association of Medical Microbiologists: www.amm.co.uk/
Association of Medical Secretaries, Practice Managers and Receptionists:
    www.amspar.co.uk/
Association of Radical Midwives: www.radmid.demon.co.uk/
Audit Commission: www.audit-commission.gov.uk/
British Association for Accident and Emergency Medicine: www.baem.org.uk/
British Association of Medical Managers: http://bamm.co.uk/awf/
British Medical Informatics Society: www.bmis.org/
British National Formulary (BNF): http://bnf.org/
British Standards Institution: www.bsi-global.com/index.xalter
British Medical Association (BMA): http://web.bma.org.uk/homepage.nsf
Centre for Health Information Quality (CHiQ): www.hfht.org/chiq/
Charity Commission: www.charity-commission.gov.uk/
Chartered Institute Of Personnel and Development: www.cipd.co.uk/
Commission for Health Improvement (CHI): www.doh.gov.uk/chi/
Dept for Education & Employment: www.dfee.gov.uk/
Department of Health: www.doh.gov.uk
Dept of Social Security: www.dss.gov.uk/
General Medical Council: www.gmc-uk.org/
GPUK.net: www.gpuk.net/
Health on the Net Foundation: www.hon.ch/HomePage/Home-Page.html
Home Office: www.homeoffice.gov.uk/
Imperial Cancer Research Fund: www.imperialcancer.co.uk/

Institute of Biomedical Sciences: www.ibms.org/
Institute of Health Record Information and Management: www.ihrim.co.uk/
International Hospital Federation: www.hospitalmanagement.net/
Joseph Rowntree Foundation: www.jrf.org.uk/home.asp
King's Fund: www.kingsfund.org.uk/
Medicines Control Agency: www.open.gov.uk/mca/mcahome.htm
National Association of Primary Care: www.primarycare.co.uk/
National Blood Service: www.blood.co.uk/welcome.htm
National Centre for Health Outcomes Development (NHSnet only): http://
    nww.nchod.nhs.uk/
New Health Network: www.newhealthnetwork.co.uk/
NHS Confederation: www.nhsconfed.net/
NHS Information Authority: www.nhsia.nhs.uk
Our Healthier Nation Report: www.ohn.gov.uk/
Pathological Society of Great Britain and Ireland: www.pathsoc.org.uk/
The Physiological Society: www.physoc.org/
Primary Health Care Group of the British Computer Society (PHCSG):
    www.phcsg.org.uk/
The Royal Pharmaceutical Society of Great Britain: www.rpsgb.org.uk/
The Royal Society of Medicine: www.rsm.ac.uk/
The Royal Statistical Society: www.rss.org.uk/
Royal College of Anaesthetists: www.rcoa.ac.uk/
Royal College of General Practitioners: www.rcgp.org.uk/
Royal College of Nursing (RCN): www.rcn.org.uk/
Royal College of Paediatrics and Child Health: www.rcpch.ac.uk/
Royal College of Physicians: www.rcplondon.ac.uk/
Royal College of Physicians of Edinburgh: www.rcpe.ac.uk/index.html
Royal College of Psychiatrists: www.rcpsych.ac.uk/
Royal College of Psychiatrists (including the College Research Unit (CRU)):
    www.rcpsych.ac.uk/cru/cru_home.htm
Royal College of Psychiatrists' Irish Division: www.irishpsychiatry.com/
Royal Pharmaceutical Society of Great Britain: www.rpsgb.org.uk/
Society for Computing and Technology in Anaesthesia: www.scata.org.uk/
Telemedicine Information Exchange (TIE): http://tie.telemed.org/
There4me: www.there4me.com/home/index.asp
UK Central Council for Nursing, Midwifery and Health Visiting (UKCC):
    www.ukcc.org.uk/; www.nmc-uk.org
UK Drug Information Pharmacist's Group (UKDIPG): www.ukdipg.org.uk/
UK NEQAS: www.ukneqas.org.uk
UK Public Health Association: www.ukpha.org.uk/
US Food and Drug Administration: www.fda.gov/opacom/hpnews.html
World Health Organization: www.who.int/

Research/academic

Centerwatch: www.centerwatch.com/main.htm
Health Services Management Centre (HSMC) – University of Birmingham:
    www.bham.ac.uk/HSMC/
Health Service Research Unit (HSRU) – University of Oxford:
    http://hsru.dphpc.ox.ac.uk/welcome.htm
Institute of Psychiatry: www.iop.kcl.ac.uk/IoP/index.stm
Medical Research Council: www.mrc.ac.uk/
National Primary Care Research & Development Centre: www.npcrdc.man.ac.uk/

UCL Clinical Research Network: www.crn.ucl.ac.uk/
University of Leicester – Greenwood Institute of Child Health: www.leicester.ac.uk/
greenwood/

Universities and colleges

Academy of Medical Royal Colleges: www.aomrc.org.uk/
College of American Pathologists: www.cap.org/
Faculty of Public Health Medicine: www.fphm.org.uk/
The Royal College of Anaesthetists: www.rcoa.ac.uk/
The Royal College of General Practitioners: www.rcgp.org.uk/
The Royal College of Nursing: www.rcn.org.uk/
The Royal College of Obstetricians and Gynaecologists: www.rcog.org.uk/
The Royal College of Ophthalmologists: www.rcophth.ac.uk/
The Royal College of Paediatrics and Child Health: www.rcpch.ac.uk/
The Royal College of Pathologists: www.rcpath.org.uk/
The Royal College of Physicians: www.rcplondon.ac.uk/
The Royal College of Psychiatrists: www.rcpsych.ac.uk/
The Royal College of Radiologists: www.rcr.ac.uk/
The Royal College of Surgeons (England): www.rcseng.ac.uk/
UCL Institute of Child Health: www.ich.ucl.ac.uk/
UCL Institute of Ophthalmology: www.ucl.ac.uk/ioo/
University of Belfast – School of Nursing and Midwifery: www.qub.ac.uk/nur/
University of Birmingham School of Medicine: http://medweb.bham.ac.uk/
med_school.html
University of Bristol – Clinical Radiology: www.bristol.ac.uk/radiology/
University of Cambridge Department of Pathology: www.path.cam.ac.uk/
University of Cambridge Department of Pharmacology: www.phar.cam.ac.uk/
University of Dundee Medical School: www.dundee.ac.uk/facmedden/
University of Edinburgh Faculty of Medicine: www.med.ed.ac.uk/
University of London St. George's Hospital Medical School: www.sghms.ac.uk/
University of Manchester – Medical Informatics Group: www.cs.man.ac.uk/mig/
University of Newcastle Faculty of Medicine: http://medical.faculty.ncl.ac.uk/
University of Sheffield Medical School: www.shef.ac.uk/uni/academic/I-M/medsch/
medsch.html
University of Southampton School of Medicine: www.som.soton.ac.uk/
University of Wales College of Medicine: www.uwcm.ac.uk/
University of Warwick – School of Postgraduate Medical Education:
www.warwick.ac.uk/fac/sci/Medical/
University of York – Centre for Health Economics: www.york.ac.uk/inst/che/
welcome.htm

Useful contact information and websites with information and data on relevant subjects

1 The link below gives you a list of every Strategic HA in England including their
   addresses and their CE name and telephone number: www.nhs.uk/england/
2 The following link takes you to a website that shows a map of every HA in England
   and the names of the PCTs in each HA: www.natpact.nhs.uk/news/
   index.php?article_request=125

3 This website lets you search for a PCT by putting in the town, giving you the CE's name and contact details: www.nhs.uk/root/localnhsservices/orgs/trust/search.asp?org=pct

4 Another page linking you to Strategic HAs and their websites (if they have one): www.info.doh.gov.uk/doh/nhsweb.nsf/Sites%20by%20Subject%20Category?OpenView&Start=1&Count=30&Expand=3.4.4.2#3.4.4.2

5 Key links in healthcare: www.info.doh.gov.uk/doh/nhsweb.nsf?Open

6 A very useful list of links for national and international medical statistics and many other things: www.lib.gla.ac.uk/Depts/MOPS/Stats/medstats.html

7 Links to all the Public Health Observatories: www.phel.gov.uk/information/websites/infosources.asp?resourcetype=Statistical

8 DoH statistics links, see also the quick links on the right-hand side of this page giving links to health surveys of England and NHS performance, hospital activity, etc.: www.doh.gov.uk/public/stats1.htm

9 Management briefing on emergency admissions with useful links: http://libraries.nelh.nhs.uk/healthmanagement/

10 National Institute for Mental Health – what is happening in mental health: www.nimhe.org.uk/

11 Salisbury Centre for Mental Health: www.scmh.org.uk/wbm23.ns4/WebLaunch/LaunchMe

12 Care trusts details: www.nhs.uk/root/localnhsservices/list_orgs.asp?ot=T__

13 Clinical databases: www.docdat.org

14 Binleys website for information about PCTs. Also you can register free and you get free access to their online maps: www.binleys.com/default.asp

15 NHS Wales with links to the informing healthcare document and many NHS Wales statisitics pages: www.wales.nhs.uk/

16 CHD Statistics: www.heartstats.org/homepage.asp

17 NHS performance ratings: www.doh.gov.uk/performanceratings/2002/summary_prtable.xls

18 Primary Care Report website and newsletter: www.primarycarereport.co.uk/

19 NAO document 'Ensuring the effective discharge of older patients from NHS acute hospitals': www.hiow.nhs.uk/board/archive/ha-028-03.pdf

20 These pages give details of government and official health-related documents (in alphabetical order) available in full text on the Web since 1997. They include Department of Health publications, Audit Commission reports, Health Select Committee reports, Health Service Ombudsman reports, National Audit Office publications and World Health Organization publications: www.herts.ac.uk/lis/subjects/health/offdoc.htm

Utilities

Acrobat Reader – PDF Viewing Software: www.adobe.com/products/acrobat/readermain.html

Adobe PDF for the Visually Impaired: http://access.adobe.com/

Download Microsoft Internet Explorer: www.microsoft.com/windows/ie/

Download Netscape Browsers: http://home.netscape.com/download/index.html

Microsoft Word/Excel Viewers: www.microsoft.com/downloads/

MUMPS – Open Source Implementation: www.sanchez-gtm.com/

Winzip: www.winzip.com/

References

Chapter 1

1 Department of Health (2002) *NHS Waiting List and Activity Figures*. DoH, London.
2 HM Treasury (2002) *Spending Review 2002: opportunity and security for all*. HMSO, London.
3 Comptroller and Auditor General NAO. HC 403 Session 2000–2001: 3 May 2001.
4 Aylin P, Bottle A, Tanna S and Jarman B (2004) Adverse events reporting in English hospital statistics. *BMJ.* **329**: 857.
5 Wanless D (2002) *Securing Our Future Health: taking a long-term view*. Final report. HM Treasury, London.

Chapter 4

1 www.statistics.gov.uk.
2 Page D, Williams P and Boyd D (1993) *Report of the Inquiry into the London Ambulance Service*. South West Thames Regional Health Authority.
3 Committee of Public Accounts (1993) *Wessex Regional Health Authority Regional Information Systems Plan*. HMSO, London. (PAC 63rd report, House of Commons, Session 1992/93.)
4 Emmerson C, Frayne C and Goodman A (2002) *How much would it cost to increase UK health spending to the European Union average?* Briefing note. Institute for Fiscal Studies, London.
5 Wanless D (2002) *Securing Our Future Health: taking a long-term view*. Final report. HM Treasury, London.

Chapter 5

1 Department of Health (1990) *Working for Patients*. HMSO, London.

Chapter 6

1 Comptroller and Auditor General (1996) *The Hospital Information Support Systems Initiative*. HC 332 1995/96.
2 Secta and Dearden (1996) *The Evaluation of the NHS Resource Management Programme in England*. University of Manchester HSMU.
3 NHS Modernisation Agency (2001) *Revision of Waiting & Booking Information (ROWBI): Draft Final Report*. www.modern.nhs.uk/rowbi/13825/rowbifinalreport2001.doc.
4 Department of Health (1992) *An Information Management and Technology Strategy for the NHS in England: IM & T strategy overview*. HMSO, London.
5 Sir John Bourne (1999) *The 1992 and 1998 Information Management & Technology Strategies of the NHS Executive*. HC 371 1998/99.
6 ERDIP (2003) *National Core Evaluation Final Report*. NHS Information Authority, London.
7 Bend J (2004) *Public Value and E-health*. Institute for Public Policy Research, London.
8 Protti D (2002) *Implementing Information for Health: even more challenging than expected?* Report for the DoH Information Policy Unit. DoH, London.

Chapter 7

1 Department of Health (2000) *The NHS Plan: a plan for investment, a plan for reform*. DoH, London.
2 HM Government. *eGovernment Strategy*.
3 Department of Health (2002) *Shifting the Balance of Power: the next steps*. DoH, London.
4 Burns F (1998) *Information for Health: an information strategy for the modern NHS*. NHS Executive, London.
5 Department of Health (2002) *Building the Information Core: implementing the NHS Plan*. DoH, London.
6 Kendall R and Lissauer L (2003) *The Future Health Worker*. IPPR, London.
7 Central Information Management Unit (2001) *e-Government Interoperability Framework V2*. CIMU, London.
8 Department of Health (1997) *The New NHS: modern, dependable*. DoH, London.
9 Department of Health (2001) *Coronary Heart Disease Information Strategy: information and IT to support the Coronary Heart Disease NSF*. DoH, London.

Chapter 8

1 General Medical Services Committee, RCGP and Joint Computing Group (1988) *The Classification of General Practice Data: final report of the GMSC-RCGP*. Joint Computing Group Technical Working Party and General Medical Services Committee, BMA, London.
2 Bates DW *et al*. (2003) Detecting adverse events using information technology. *J Am Med Inform Assoc*. **10**(2): 115–18.

Chapter 10

1 Brennan S (2002) Sir John Pattison talks to Sean Brennan. *Br J Healthcare Comput Info Manage*. **19**(7): 2–5.

Chapter 13

1 Bates DW *et al*. (1999) A randomized trial of a computer-based intervention to reduce utilization of redundant laboratory tests. *Am J Med*. **106**(2): 144–50.
2 Chin HL and Wallace P (1999) Embedding guidelines into direct physician order entry: simple methods, powerful results. *Proc AMIA Annu Symp*. 221–5.
3 van Wijk MA *et al*. (2001) Assessment of decision support for blood test ordering in primary care. A randomised trial. *Annals of Internal Medicine*. **134**: 274–81.
4 Arrowe Park Hospital, Wirral and Queens Hospital, Burton (1998) *EPR Demonstrator Site: final report*. NHS Executive, Leeds.
5 Bates DW and Gawande AA (2003) Improving safety with information technology. *N Engl J Med*. **348**(25): 2526–34.
6 Kohn L, Corrigan J and Donaldson M (eds) (2000) *To Err is Human: building a safer health system*. National Academy Press, Washington, DC.
7 Dean B, Schachter M, Vincent C and Barber N (2002) Prescribing errors in hospital inpatients: their incidence and clinical significance. *Qual Saf Health Care*. **11**: 340–4.
8 Farrar K (2004) Minimising adverse drug events. *Public Service Review: Central Government*. **Spring**: 48–9.
9 Audit Commission (2001) *A Spoonful of Sugar: medicines management in NHS hospitals*. Audit Commission Report. Audit Commission, London.
10 Audit Commission (1994) *A Prescription for Improvement: towards more rational prescribing in general practice*. Audit Commission, London.

11 Bowden JE (1993) Reissuing patients' medicines: a step to seamless care. *Pharm J.* **251**: 356.
12 Dobrzanski S and Reidy F (1993) The pharmacist as a discharge medication planner in surgical patients. *Pharm J.* HS53–HS56.
13 Bates DW, Leape LL, Cullen DJ, Laird N *et al.* (1998) Effect of computerized physician order entry and a team intervention on prevention of serious medication errors. *JAMA.* **280**: 1311–16.
14 Hughes D, Farrar KT and Slee A (2001) The trials and tribulations of electronic prescribing. *Hospital Prescriber Europe.* **1**: 74–6.
15 Chester MI and Zilz DA (1989) Effects of bar coding on a pharmacy stock replenishment system. *Am J Hosp Pharm.* **46**: 1380–5.
16 Slee A, Farrar K and Hughes D (2002) The benefits of automation. *Pharm J.* **268**: 437–8.
17 Bates DW (2000) Using information to reduce rates of medication errors in hospitals. *BMJ.* **320**: 788–91.
18 Barker A (2004) Electronic prescribing must be introduced for the right reasons. *Pharm J.* **273**: 20.
19 West Suffolk Presentation – personal communication.
20 Norfolk & Norwich Radiology Department – personal communication.
21 Kings College Hospital – personal communication.
22 Department of Health (2000) *The NHS Plan: a plan for investment, a plan for reform.* DoH, London (Sections 4.19 and 4.20).
23 Strickland N (1996) Some cost-benefit considerations for PACS: a radiological perspective. *Br J Radiol.* **69**: 1089–98; Huang HK (2003) *Comput Med Imaging Graph.* **27**(2–3): 241–53.
24 Bryan S, Weatherburn G, Watkins J, Keen J, Muris N and Buxton M (1998) *The Evaluation of a Hospital-Wide Picture Archiving and Communication System (PACS).* Report to the Department of Health of the Brunel Evaluation of the Hammersmith PACS System. DoH, London.
25 PACS and Teleradiology Group Meeting.
26 Derbyshire CMHT (2004) The Improvement Network. www.tin.nhs.uk/welcome/good-news-stories/derbyshire-cmht
27 Templeton SK (2002) Forget the grapes and the flowers, virtual visiting is the way forward. *Sunday Herald.* 3 Feb, p. 6.
28 Cappuccio FP, Kerry SM, Forbes L and Donald A (2004) Blood pressure control by home monitoring: meta-analysis of randomised trials. *BMJ.* **329**: 145.

Chapter 14

1 HM Government (2001) *Health and Social Care Act.* HMSO, London.
2 Kennedy I (2001) *The Report of the Public Inquiry into Children's Heart Surgery at the Bristol Royal Infirmary, 1984–1995: learning from Bristol.* HMSO, London.
3 Health Which/NPfIT (2003) *The Public View on Electronic Health Records.* Health Which/NPfIT, www.dh.gov.uk/assetRoot/04/05/50/46/04055046.pdf

Chapter 15

1 Bates DW *et al.* (2003) Detecting adverse events using information technology. *J Am Med Inform Assoc.* **10**(2): 115–18.
2 Bates DW *et al.* (1999) A randomized trial of a computer-based intervention to reduce utilization of redundant laboratory tests. *Am J Med.* **106**(2): 144–50.
3 Collins T with Bicknell D (1997) *Crash: Ten easy ways to avoid a computer disaster.* Simon & Schuster, New York.
4 Maurer R (1996) *Beyond the Wall of Resistance: Unconventional strategies that build support for change.* Bard Press, Austin, TX.

Index

Page numbers in *italics* refer to tables or figures.